Hand Acupuncture Therapy

Chief - Editor: Zhao Xin

Editor: Qiao Jinlin, Li Guohua

Academy Press [Xue Yuan]

First Edition 1997

ISBN7 − 5077 − 1375 − X

Hand Acupuncture Therapy

Chief − Editor: Zhao Xin

Editor: Qiao Jinlin, Li Guohua

Published by

Academy Press [Xue Yuan]

11 Wanshoulu Xijie, Beijing 100036, China

Distributed by

China International Book Trading Corporation

35 Chegongzhuang Xilu, Beijing 100044, China

P. O. Box 399, Beijing, China

Printed in the People's Republic of China

Preface

The hand acupuncture therapy as a treatment with acupuncture and moxibustion applied to hand for general diseases of the body was in vogue in recent years. Human hand is closely related to internal organs, meridians, qi and blood. The acupoints of **14** meridians and extra acupoints discovered in past successive dynasties and the effective spots developed in modern times are distributed on the hand. In this book the acupoints and their usage for diseases of different medical branches were discussed as a reference for clinical application of acupuncture physicians and amateurs.

Chief — Editor

Contents

Part I   Points of Hand Acupuncture

Chapter One   Points of the Meridians ············ (1)

Part II   Clinical Therapy

Part I Points of Hand Acupuncture

Chapter One
Points of the Meridians

Yújì(LU10)
Location   In the depression proximal to the first metacarpophalangeal point, on the radial side of the midpoint of the first metacarpal bone, and on the junction of the dorsal and palmar skin.

Indications   fever, sore throat, cough with abundant expectoration, dyspnea or shortness of breath, distention of the chest.

Shàoshāng(LU11)
Location   On the radial side of the distal segment of the thumb, 0.1 *cun* from the corner of the fingernail.

Indications   Nosebleed, pharyngitis or tonsillitis, apoplexy with unconsciousness, cough and dyspnea.

Shāngyáng(LI1)

Location　On the radial side of the distal segment of the index finger, 0.1 *cun* from the corner of the nail.

Indications　Tinnitus, deafness, dry mouth, swelling of the cheek(s), optic atrophy, syndrome involving the head, face or throat, fever.

Èrjiān(LI2)

Location　In the depression of the radial side, distal to the second metacarpophalangeal joint when a loose fist is made.

Indications　toothache, nosebleed, blurring of vision, pharyngitis or tonsillitis, fever.

Sānjiān(LI3)

Location　In the depression of the radial side, proximal to the second metacarpophalangeal joint when a loose fist is made.

Indications　Dental caries, eye pain, fever, sore throat.

Hégǔ(LI4)

Location　On the dorsum of the hand, between the first and second metacarpal bones, and on the radial side of the midpoint of the second metacarpal bone.

Indications　headache, deviation of the eye and mouth, toothache, swelling of the cheek(s), facial spasms, nasal obstruction, fever, flaccidity of hand(s).

Yángxī(LI5)

Location At the radial end of the crease of the wrist, in the depression between the tendons of the short extensor and long extensor muscles of the thumb when the thumb is tilted upward.

Indications congestion of conjunctiva and swelling pain of eye(s), delirious speech.

Shàofǔ(HT8)

Location In the palm, between the fourth and fifth metacarpal bones, at the part of the palm touching the tip of the little finger when a fist is made.

Indications feverish sensation of the palms, difficulty in urination, malaria, glossodynia and glossoncus, brachialgia, pain in the elbow.

Shàochōng(HT9)

Location On the radial side of the distal segment of the little finger, 0.1 *cun* from the corner of the nail.

Indications fever, restlessness, epigastric pain, precordial pain, shortness of breath.

Shàozé(SI1)

Location On the ulnar side of the distal segment of the little finger, 0.1 *cun* from the corner of the nail.

Indications   Laryngitis, apoplexy, galactostasis, cataract, fever with unconsciousness.

Qiángǔ(SI2)

Location   At the junction of the dorsal and ventral skin along the ulnar border of the hand, at the ulnar end of the crease of the fifth metacarpophalangeal joint when a loose fist is made.

Indications   Tinnitus, fever with no perspiration, dizziness, headache accompanied with distending sensation, restlessness.

Hòuxī(SI3)

Location   At the junction of the dorsal and palmar skin along the ulnar border of the hand, at the ulnar end of the distal palmar crease, proximal to the fifth metacarpophalangeal joint when a hollow fist is made.

Indications   Stiff pain of the nape, omalgia and brachialgia, pain in the elbow, tinnitus and deafness, mania.

Wàngǔ(SI4)

Location   On the ulnar border of the hand, in the depression between the proximal end of the fifth metacarpal bone and hamate bone, and at the junction of the dorsal and palmar skin.

Indications   Jaundice, swelling of the cheek(s) with difficulty in opening mouth, fever with unconsciousness.

Láogōng(PC8)

Location   At the center of the palm, between the second and third metacarpal bones, but close to the latter, and in the part touching the tip of the middle finger when a fist is made.

Indications   Fever, vomiting, nosebleed, hiccup, mania or depression, unconsciousness.

Zhōngchōng(PC9)

Location   At the center of the tip of the middle finger.

Indications   Precordial pain or epigastric pain, feverish sensation in the palms and soles, fever with no perspiration, apoplexy.

Guānchōng(SJ1)

Location   On the ulnar side of the distal segment of the fourth finger, 0.1 *cun* from the corner of the nail.

Indications   Laryngitis, tonsillitis, restlessness, precordial pain or epigastric pain, distention in the chest. curled - up tongue.

Yèmén(SJ2)

Location   On the dorsum of the hand, between the fourth and fifth fingers, at the junction of the red and white skin, proximal to the margin of the web.

Indications   Congestion of the conjunctiva, tinnitus and deafness, sore throat, fever.

Zhōngzhǔ(SJ3)

Location   On the dorsum of the hand, proximal to the fourth metacarpophalangeal joint, in the depression between the fourth and fifth metacarpal bones.

Indications   Fever with no perspiration, headache, deafness, cataract.

Yángchí(SJ4)

Location   At the midpoint of the dorsal crease of the wrist, in the depression on the ulnar side of the tendon of the extensor muscle of the fingers.

Indications   Thirst due to diabetes, sore throat, fever, carpal pain.

Chapter Two
Extra Points

Extra Points on the Hand

Dàgǔkōng(EX – UE5)
Location On the dorsal side o the thumb, at the center of the interphalangeal joint.

Indications Eye diseases, stomachache, vomiting.

Xiǎogǔkōng(EX – UE6)
Location On the dorsal side of the little finger, at the center of the proximal interphalangeal joint.

Indications Fever, eye diseases. Moxibustion is applied.

Yāotòngdiǎn(EX – UE7)
Location Two points on the dorsum of each hand, between the first and second and between the third and fourth

metacarpal bones, and at the midpoint between the dorsal crease of the wrist and the metacarpophalangeal joint.

Indications   Lumbago.

Wàiláogōng(EX － UE8)

Location   On the dorsum of the hand, between the second and third metacarpal bones, and 0.5 *cun* proximal to the metacarpophalangeal joint.

Indications   Epigastric pain, pain in the abdomen.

Bāxié(EX － UE9)

Location   Four points on the dorsum of each hand, at the junction of the red and white skin proximal to the margin of the webs between each two of the five fingers of a hand.

Indications   Fever, pains.

Sìfèng(EX － UE10)

Location   Four points on each hand, on the palmar side of the second to fifth fingers and at the center of the proximal interphalangeal joints.

Indications   Malnutrition due to improper feeding. Punctured with three － edged needle.

Shíxuān(EX – UE11)

Location   Ten points on both hands, at the tips of the 10 fingers, 0.1 *cun* from the free margin of the nails.

Indications   Fever, hypertension. Generally applied for emergent diseases.

Chapter Three

Some New Points of Hand Acupuncture

1. Huáidiǎn

Location   On the red – white border, radial side of the metacarpophalangeal joint of the thumb.

Indications   Sprain of ankle joint with pain.

2. Xiōngdiǎn

Location   On the red – white border, radial side of the pollical joint.

Indications   Chest pain, vomiting, diarrhea, epilepsy.

3. Yǎndiǎn

Location   On the red – white border, ulnar side

of the pollical joint.

Indications   Ophthalmic diseases, such as conjunctival congestion, ophthalmalgia, blurred vision, hordeolum, optic atrophy.

4. Jiāndiǎn

Location   On the red − white border, radial side of the metacarpophalangeal joint of the index finger.

Indications   Sprain of the shoulder joint, omalgia, scapulohumeral periarthritis.

5. Qiántóudiǎn

Location   On the red − white border, radial side of the first metacarpophalangeal joint of the index finger.

Indications   Headache, gastric pain, vomiting, abdominal pain, diarrhea, appendicitis, omalgia, toothache.

6. Tóudǐngdiǎn

Location   On the red − white border, radial side of the first middle finger joint.

Indications   Parietal headache, dysmenorrhea.

7. Piāntóudiǎn

Location On the red – white border, ulnar side of the first ring finger joint.

Indications Migraine, intercostal neuralgia.

8. Huìyīndiǎn

Location On the red – white border, radial side of the first little finger joint.

Indications Dysmenorrhea, morbid vaginal discharge, pain in the perineum.

9. Hòutóudiǎn

Location On the red – white border, ulnar side of the first little finger joint.

Indications Headache in the occiput, sore – throat, tonsillitis, stiffness of the nape, pain in the shoulder and arm, pain in the cheek.

10. Jǐzhùdiǎn

Location On the red – white border, ulnar side of the metacarpophalangeal joint of the little finger.

Indications Lumbago, sprain of the lumbar joint, prolapse of lumbar intervertebral disc, coccyalgia and sacral pain, tinnitus, stuffy nose.

11. Zuògǔshénjīngdiǎn

Location   On the dorsum of the hand, between the fourth and fifth metacarpophalangeal joints, proximal to the fourth.

Indications   Sciatica, pain in the hip joint and pygalgia.

12. Yānhóudiǎn

Location   On the dorsum of the hand, between the third and fourth metacarpophalangeal joints, proximal to the third.

Indications   Acute tonsillitis, pharyngitis and laryngitis.

13. Tóuxiàngdiǎn

Location   On the dorsum of the hand, between the second and third metacarpophalangeal joints, proximal to the second.

Indications   Stiff neck or sprain of the nape.

14. Wèichángtòngdiǎn

Location   On the palm, at the midpoint between **Láogōng**(PC8) and **Dàlíng**(PC7).

Indications   Chronic gastritis, peptic ulcer, apepsia.

15. Kéchuǎndiǎn

Location   On the palm, ulnar side of the second metacarpophalangeal joint.

Indications   Bronchitis, cough.

16. Xiàochuǎndiǎn

Location   On the palm, between the fourth and fifth metacarpophalangeal joints.

Indications   Asthma.

17. Zúgēntòngdiǎn

Location   At the midpoint between Weichang-tongdian and **Dàlíng(PC7)**.

Indications   Painful heels.

18. Shēngyàdiǎn

Location   At the midpoint of the dorsal crease of the wrist.

Indications   Hypotension.

19. È'nìdiǎn

Location　On the dorsal side of middle finger, at the midpoint of crease of the second joint.

Indications　Hiccough.

20. Tuìrèdiǎn

Location　On the dorsum of the hand, radial to the middle finger, at the junction of the red and white skin, proximal to the web.

Indications　Fever, eye diseases.

21. Fùxièdiǎn

Location　On the dorsum of the hand, 1 *cun* proximal to the midpoint between the third and fourth metacarpophalangeal joints.

Indications　Diarrhea.

22. Nǜèjídiǎn

Location　On the junction between the first metacarpal bone and carpal joint, radial to the margin of the thenar.

Indications　Malaria.

23. Biǎntáotǐdiǎn

Location　On the palm, at the midpoint of the ulnar side of the first metacarpal bone.

Indications　Tonsillitis, laryngitis.

24. Jíjiùdiǎn

Location　On the distal segment of the middle finger, at the midpoint of the tip, 0.2 *cun* from the corner of the nail.

Indications　Coma.

25. Dìngjīngdiǎn

Location　On the palm, at the midpoint of the junction between the thenar and hypothenar.

Indications　Convulsion.

26. Pídiǎn

Location　On the palmar side of the thumb, at the midpoint of the crease between the distal and proximal segments.

Indications　Digestive diseases, cancer.

27. Xiǎochángdiǎn

Location   On the palmar side of the index, at the midpoint of the crease between the proximal and middle segments.

Indications   Diseases affecting small intestine.

28. Dàchángdiǎn

Location   On the palmar side of the index, at the midpoint of the crease between the distal and middle segments.

Indications   Diseases affecting large intestine.

29. Sānjiāodiǎn

Location   On the palmar side of the middle finger, at the midpoint of the crease between the proximal and middle segments.

Indications   Diseases affecting chest, abdomen, and pelvic cavity.

30. Xīndiǎn

Location   On the palmar side of the middle finger, at the midpoint of the crease between the distal and middle segments.

Indications   Cardiovascular diseases.

31. Gāndiǎn
Location   On the palmar side of the ring finger, at the midpoint of the crease between the proximal and middle segments.

Indications   Hepatocystic diseases.

32. Fèidiǎn
Location   On the palmar side of the ring finger, at the midpoint of the crease between the distal and middle segments.

Indications   Respiratory diseases.

33. Mìngméndiǎn
Location   On the palmar side of the little finger, at the midpoint of the crease between the proximal and middle segments.

Indications   Diseases affecting the reproductive system.

34. Shèndiǎn
Location   On the palmar side of the little finger,

at the midpoint of the crease between the distal and middle segments.

Indications   Enuresis, frequency of urination, diseases affecting the urinary system.

Part II   Clinical Therapy

Chapter One
Internal Diseases

Cerebrovascular Accidents

Cerebrovascular accident, or stroke, is a focal neurologic disorder due to a pathologic process in a blood vessel. In most cases the onset is abrupt and evolution rapid, and symptoms reach a peak within seconds, minutes or hours. Partial or complete recovery may occur over a period of hours to months.

Occlusion of a cerebral artery by thrombosis or embolism results in a cerebral infarction with its associated clinical effects. Other conditions may on occasion also produce cerebral infarction and thus may be confused with cerebral arteritis, systemic hypotension, reactions to cerebral angiography, and transient cerebral ischemia.

Cerebral hemorrhage is usually caused by rupture of an

arteriosclerotic cerebral vessel. Subarachnoid hemorrhage is usually due to rupture of a congenitally weak blood vessel or aneurysm.

Transient cerebral ischemia may also occur without producing a cerebral infarction. Premonitory recurrent focal cerebral ischemic attacks may occur and are apt to be in a repetitive pattern in a given case. Attack may last for 10 seconds to one hour, but the average duration is 2 to 10 minutes. As many as several hundred such attacks may occur. In some instances of transient ischemia, the neurologic deficit may last up to 20 hours.

Narrowing of the extracranial arteries (particularly the internal carotid artery at its origin in the neck and, in some cases, the intrathoracic arteries) by arteriosclerotic patches has been incriminated in a significant number of cases of transient cerebral ischemias and infarction.

In traditional Chinese medicine, the disease is considered to be caused by stirring wind arising from hyperactivity of Yang in the liver which results from exasperation or agitation accompanied with disturbance of the Zang − fu organs. Qi and blood imbalance of Yin and Yang and dysfunction of the channels and collaterals. Another factor is endogenous wind caused by phlegm − heat after over − indulgence in alcohol and fatty diet.

Clinical Manifestations

Early phase. Variable degrees and types occur. The onset may be violent, with the patient falling to the ground and lying inert like a person in deep sleep, with flushed, face, stertorous or Cheyne – stroke respirations, full and slow pulse, and one arm and leg usually flaccid. Death may occur in a few hours or days. Lesser grades of stroke may consist of slight derangement of speech, thought, motion, sensation, or vision. Consciousness need not be altered. Symptoms may last seconds to minutes or longer or may persist unremittingly for an indefinite period. Some degree of recovery is usual.

Premonitory symptoms may include headache, dizziness, drowsiness, and mental confusion. Focal premonitory symptoms are more likely to occur with thrombosis.

Generalized neurologic signs are most common with cerebral hemorrhage and include fever, headache, vomiting, convulsion, and coma. Nuchal rigidity is frequent with subarachnoid hemorrhage or intracerebral hemorrhage. Mental changes are commonly noted in the period following a stroke and may include confusion, disorientation and memory defects.

Main Points of Diagnosis

1. Sudden onset of neurologic complaints varying from focal motor or hypesthesia and speech defects to profound coma.

2. May be associated with vomiting, convulsions or headaches.

3. Nuchal rigidity is frequently found.

Differential Diagnosis and Treatment

1) Syndrome due to attack at internal organs

This syndrome can be further divided into excessive and deficient types.

(1) Excessive syndrome

Yang – excessive syndrome   The patients may suddenly fall down and lose consciousness, and they may suffer from locked jaw, clenched hands, flushed face, deep breath with wheezing noise in the throat due to abundant expectoration. The pulse is wiry, rolling and rapid and the tongue coating is yellow and greasy.

Therapeutic principle   To open orifices of sense organs and discharge phlegm, and to suppress hyperactivity of liver and stop wind blow.

Principal acupoints   **Shuǐgōu** (**DU26**),   **Yǒngquán** (**KI1**), **Láogōng**(**PC8**), **Jíjiùdiǎn**.

Supplemental acupoints   **Gāndiǎn**, **Taichong** (**LR 3**), and **Nèiguān**(**PC6**).

According to the clinical manifestation, the patent herbal pills may be administered to treat deep coma. Zixuedan, Zhibao dan and Angong Niuhuang wan are commonly administered.

Yin - excessive syndrome   The patients are quiet without restlessness, and they also suffer from pale complexion, cyanotic lips, cold limbs and accumulation of phlegm and saliva. The tongue coating is white, slippery and greasy and the pulse is deep, wiry and rolling.

Therapeutic principle   To open orifices of sense organs with pungent and warm herbs and to resolve phlegm and release stasis in the collateral.

Principal acupoints   **Gāndiǎn**, **Shàoshāng**(**LU11**).

Supplemental acupoints   **Zhōngchōng** (**PC9**), **Yújì** (**LU10**), **Shāngyáng**(**LI1**) and **Láogōng**(**PC8**).

(2) Deficient syndrome   The patients may suffer from stroke and coma with eyes closed, mouth opened, fingers separated from each other, cold limbs, snoring, shallow breath and oily sweat. The tongue is paralytic and the pulse is indistinct.

Principal acupoints   **Láogōng**(**PC8**) and **Bāxié**(**EX** −

UE9).

Supplemental acupoints   Tàixī(KI3), Gāndiǎn, Hòuxī (SI3) and Yújì(LU10).

2) Syndrome due to attack at meridians

The patients may suffer from hemiplegia, deviation of mouth and eye, dizziness, vertigo and dysphasia. The pulse is wiry and rolling or deep and thready.

Therapeutic principle   To resolve phlegm and release stasis in the collateral.

Principal acupoints   Bāxié(EX – UE9), Hégǔ(LI4).

Supplemental acupoints   Shàoshāng (LU11), Shāngyáng(LI1), Zhōngchōng(PC9), Guānchōng(SJ1), Shàochōng(HT9), Shàozé(SI1) and Wàngǔ(SI4). Reducing method of acupuncture is applied to the normal side first; and then reinforcing method is applied to the diseased side.

Note   Hand acupuncture therapy can only be applied as a supplemental treatment to the patient suffering from apoplexy.

Vertigo

Vertigo is a common clinical symptom of some diseases, such as air sickness and sea sickness with blurred vision and a rotating sensation.

Etiology and Pathogenesis

The pathogenic organs of vertigo are liver and kidney and the pathogenic factor is deficiency or excessiveness of body. In deficient type, the kidney *yin* is deficient, which is caused by mental depression. The liver is an organ with the nature of wind and wood. Its anatomical structures are *yin* in nature; but its physiological function is *yang* in nature. The liver and kidney are both located in Xiajiao (lower energizer) and the liver is nourished by the kidney water (Yin). Once the kidney *yin* is deficient, the liver *yang* may become hyperactive to produce endogenous wind pathogen to attack the brain. The worriment and tiredness may damage heart and spleen. If the heart is damaged, ying (nutrient material) will be insufficient; and if the spleen is damaged, it can not produce sufficient *qi* and blood, the head and eyes can not obtain enough nutrients supplied from spleen. The excessive sexual life may cause deficiency of kidney essence *yin* and the brain will be depleted of nutrients because of the poor supply of essence from kidney. The dampness and phlegm accumulated in body may be transferred into *fire* pathogen and the conjugated phlegm and *fire* may be transported upward to attack the head and eyes. The upward transportation of clear *yang* is blocked by the accumulated dampness pathogen, but the turbid *yin* may take the place of clear *yang* and ascend up to attack the head and eyes.

Differential Diagnosis and Treatment

1) Excessiveness of liver *yang*

The patients may suffer from vertigo, headache, flushed face, tinnitus, palpitation of heart, insomnia, dreaminess, numbness of limbs and high irritability and angry. The tongue proper is red and the pulse is wiry and thready.

Therapeutic principle   To suppress hyperactivity of liver and control exacerbation of *yang*.

Principal acupoints   **Gāndiǎn, Láogōng (PC8)** and **Bǎihuì(DU20)**.

Supplemental acupoints **Hégǔ(LI4), Tàichōng(LR3)** and **Sānjiāodiǎn**.

2) Deficiency of essence

The patients may suffer from vertigo to cause falling down, sallow complexion, depressed spirit, shortness of breath, no desire to speak, palpitation of heart, insomnia, tinnitus and empty feeling in brain. The tongue proper is pale with thin coating and the pulse is thready and weak.

Therapeutic principle To tonify essence.

Principal acupoints **Shèndiǎn, Tàixī (KI3)** and **Yǒngquán(KI1)**.

Supplemental acupoints **Hégǔ (LI4), Tàichōng (LR3), Xīndiǎn** and **Sānjiāodiǎn**.

3) Upward attack of conjugated phlegm and *fire* pathogen

The patients may suffer from vertigo, pain and distension of head, annoyance, palpitation of heart, bitter taste in mouth and stomach distress. The tongue proper is red with yellow and greasy coating and the pulse is rolling and rapid or wiry and rolling.

Therapeutic principle To clear heat and resolve phlegm.

Principal acupoints **Shàoshāng (LU11), Shāngyáng (LI1)** and **Sānjiāodiǎn**.

Supplemental acupoints **Yèmén(SJ2), Yángchí(SJ4)**, and **Láogōng(PC8)**.

4) Obstruction of turbid fluid pathogen in spleen and stomach

The patients may suffer from vertigo, fullness in chest and upper abdomen, nausea and heaviness of head. The tongue proper is pale with white greasy coating and the pulse is soft and rolling.

Therapeutic principle   To strengthen spleen and resolve dampness and turbid fluid pathogen.

Principal acupoints   **Hégǔ** (**LI**4), **Pídiǎn** and **Sānjiāodiǎn**.

Supplemental acupoints   **Tàiyuān(LU9)** and **Bāxié(EX – UE9)**.

The moxibustion with atractylodes may be applied at **Pídiǎn** and **Sānjiāodiǎn** with moxa cones of a pit of date in size changed for 5 times.

A thin magnetic flat may be applied to **Yǒngquán(KI1)** and fixed with adhesive plaster to treat vertigo and hypertension. **Yángchí(SJ4)** may also be used for this treatment.

Hypertension

An elevated arterial pressure is probably the more important public health problem in developed countries − − being common, asymptomatic, readily detectable, usually easily treatable, and often leading to lethal complications if left untreated. Although our understanding of the pathophysiology of an elevated arterial pressure has increased, in 90 to 95 percent of cases the etiology (and thus potentially the prevention or cure)is still unknown.

Definition

Since there is no dividing line between normal and high blood pressure but also systolic pressure, age, sex, and race. For example, patients with a diastolic pressure greater than 12.0 kPa (90 mmHg) will have a significant reduction in morbidity and mortality with adequate therapy. These , then, are patients who have hypertension and who should be considered for treatment.

The level of systolic pressure is important in assessing arterial pressures influence on cardiovascular morbidity . Males with normal diastolic pressures (< 10. 9 kPa, 82 mmHg), but elevated systolic pressures (> 21 kPa, 158 mmHg) have a 2.5 fold increase in their cardiovascular mortality rates when compared with individuals with similar diastolic pressures but whose systolic pressures are normal (< 17.3 kPa, 130 mmHg).

Other significant factors which modify blood pressures influence on the frequency of morbid cardiovascular events are age, race, and sex with young black males being most adversely affected by hypertension.

Thus, even though in an adult hypertension is usually defined as a pressure greater than or equal to 20.0/12.0 kPa (150/90 mmHg), in men under 45 years of a pressure greater than or equal to 17.3/12.0 kPa (130/90 mmHg) may be elevated.

Individuals can be classified as being normotensive if arterial pressure is less than the levels noted above and as having destined hypertension if the diastolic pressure always exceeds these levels. Arterial pressure fluctuates in most persons, whether they are normotensive or hypertensive. Those who are classified as having labile hypertension are patients who sometimes but not always have arterial pressures within the hypertensive range. These patients are often considered to have borderline hypertension.

Sustained hypertension can become accelerated or enter malignant phase. Though a patient with malignant hypertension often has a blood pressure above 26.6/18.7 kPa (200/140 mmHg), it is papilledema, usually accompanied by retinal hemorrhages and exudates, and not the absolute pressure level, that defines this condition. Accelerated hypertension signifies a significant recent increase over previous hypertensive levels associated with evidence of vascular damage on funduscopic examination but without papilledema.

In 1978, World Health Organization (WHO) determined;

1. Normal blood pressure: Systolic pressure≤18.7Kpa (140mmHg), diastolic≤12.0 kPa(90 mmHg).

2. Hypertension: Systolic pressure ≥21.3 kPa (160 mmHg) or diastolic pressure≥12.6 kPa (95 mmHg). 3. Borderline hypertension: Systolic pressure 18.9~21.1 kPa (141~159 mmHg), diastolic pressure 12.1~12.5 kPa (91 ~94 mmHg).

Etiology

The cause of elevated arterial pressure is unknown in most cases. There are no available data to define the frequency of secondary hypertension in the general population, although in middle $--$ aged males it has been reported to be 6 percent. On the other hand , in referral centers where patients undergo an extensive evaluation, it has been reported to be as high as 35 percent.

Essential Hypertension   Patients with arterial hypertension and no definable cause are said to have primary, essential, or idiopathic hypertension. By definition, the underlying mechanism(s) is unknown; however, the kidney probably plays a central role.

1. Heredity   Genetic factors have long been assumed to be important in the genesis of hypertension . One approach has been to assess the correlation of blood pressures within familial aggregation). From these studies the minimum size of the genetic factor can be expressed by a correlation coefficient of approximately 0.2.

2. Environment   A number of environmental factors have been specifically implicated in the development of hypertension including salt intake, obesity, occupation, family size, and crowding. These factors have all been assumed to be important in the increase in blood pressure with age in more affluent societies, in contrast to the decline in blood pressure with age in more primitive cultures. Indeed, even the familial aggregation of blood pressure has been suggested as being related, at least in part, to environmental rather than genetic factors. However, since adopted children do not demonstrate familial aggregation of blood pressure, this phe-

nomenon is probably almost entirely the result of genetic factors.

3. Factors modifying the course of essential hypertension Age, race, sex, smoking, serum cholesterol, glucose intolerance, weight, and perhaps renin activity may all alter the prognosis of this disease.

Secondary Hypertension In only a small minority of patients with an elevated arterial pressure can a specific cause be identified. Nearly all the secondary forms are related to an alteration in hormone secretion and /or renal function.

1. Renal hypertension Hypertension produced by renal disease is the result of either (1) a derangement in the renal handling of sodium and fluids leading to volume expansion or (2) an alteration in renal secretion of vasoactive materials resulting in a systemic or local change in arteriolar tone. A simple explanation for renal vascular hypertension is that decreased perfusion of renal tissue due to stenosis of a main or branch renal artery activates the vasoconstriction, by stimulation of aldosterone secretion with resultant sodium retention, and/or by stimulating the adrenergic nervous system. In actual practice only about one half of patients with renovascular hypertension have elevated absolute levels of renin activity in peripheral plasma , although when renin measurements are referenced against an index of sodium balance, a much higher fraction has inappropriately high values.

A recently described form of renal hypertension results

from the excess secretion of renin by juxtaglomerular cell tumors or nephroblastomas. The initial presentation has been similar to that of hyperaldosteronism with hypertension, hypokalemia, and overproduction of aldosterone. However, on contrast to primary aldosteronism, peripheral renal activity is elevated instead of subnormal. This disease can be distinguished from other form of secondary aldosteronism by the presence of normal renal function and with unilateral increases internal vein renin concentration without a renal artery lesion.

2. Endocrine hypertension (adrenal hypertension)

Hypertension is a feature of a variety of adrenal cortical abnormalities. In primary aldosteronism there is a clear relationship between the aldosterone − induced, sodium retention and the hypertension. Normal individuals given aldosterone develop hypertension only if they also ingest sodium. Since aldosterone causes sodium retention by stimulating renal tubular exchange of sodium for potassium, hypokalemia is a prominent feature in mist patients with primary aldosteronism, and the measurement of serum potassium provides a simple screening test, The effect of sodium retention and volume expansion in chronically suppressing plasma renin activity is critically important for the definitive diagnosis. In most clinical situations plasma renin activity and plasma or urinary aldosterone levels parallel each other, but on patients with primary aldosteronism, aldosterone levels are high and relatively fixed because of autonomous aldosterone secretion, while plasma renin activity levels are suppressed and respond sluggishly to sodium deletion. Primary aldosteronism may be secondary either to a tumor or bilateral adrenal hyperplasia. It is important to distinguish between these two conditions preoperatively, as usually the hypertension in the latter is not modified by operation.

The most common cause of endocrine hypertension is that resulting from the use of estrogen – containing oral contraceptives. Indeed, this may be the most common form of secondary hypertension. The mechanism producing the hypertension is likely to be secondary to activation of the renin – angiotensin – aldosterone system.

3. Coarctation of the aorta   The hypertension associated with coarctation may be caused by the constriction itself, or perhaps by the changes in the renal circulation which result in an unusual form of renal arterial hypertension. The diagnosis of coarctation is usually evident from physical examination and routine x – ray findings.

4. Low – renin essential hypertension   Approximately 20 percent of patients who by all other criteria have essential hypertension have suppressed plasma renin activity. Recent studies have suggested that many of these patients have an increased sensitivity to angiotensin 2 which may be the underlying mechanism: Since this altered sensitivity has been reported even in patients with normal renin hypertension, it

is likely that patients with low – renin hypertension are not a distinct subset but rather form part of a continuum of patients with essential hypertension.

5. High – renin essential hypertension   Approximately 15 percent of patients with essential hypertension have plasma renin levels elevated above the normal range. It has been suggested that plasma renin plays an important role in the pathogenesis of the elevated blood pressure in these patients. However, most studies have documented that saralasin significantly reduces blood pressure in less than half of these patients. This has led some investigators to postulate that the elevated renin levels and blood pressure may both be secondary to an increased activity of the adrenergic system. It has been proposed that, in those patients with angiotensin – dependent high – renin hypertension whose arterial pressures are lowered by saralasin, the mechanism responsible for the increased renin and, therefore, the hypertension is a compensatory one secondary to a decreased adrenal responsiveness to angiotensin Ⅱ.

Effects of Hypertension   For nearly 70 years it has been known that patients with hypertension die prematurely. The most common cause of death is heart disease , with strokes and renal failure also frequently occurring, particularly in those with significant retinopathy.

Effects on Heart   Cardiac compensation for the excessive work load imposed by increased systemic pressure is at first sustained by left ventricular hypertrophy. Ultimately, the function of this chamber deteriorates, it dilates, and the symptoms and signs of heart failure appear. Angina pectoris may also occur because of accelerated coronary arterial disease and /or increased myocardial oxygen requirements as a consequence of the increased myocardial mass, which exceeds the capacity of the coronary circulation. On physical examination the heart is enlarged and has a prominent left ventricular impulse. The sound of aortic closure is accentuated, and there may be a faint murmur of aortic regurgitation. Presystolic (atrial, fourth) heart sounds appear frequently on hypertensive heart disease, and a protodiastolic (ventricular, third heart) sound or summation gallop rhythm may be present. Electrocardiographic changes of left ventricular hypertrophy are common; evidence of ischemia or infarction may be observed late in the disease. The majority of deaths due to hypertension result from myocardial infarction or congestive heart failure.

Neurologic Effects   The neurologic effects of long – standing hypertension may be divided into retinal and central nervous system changes. Because the retina is the only tissue in which the arteries and arterioles can be examined directly, repeated ophthalmoscopic examination provides the opportunity to observe the progress of the vascular effects of hypertension. The Keith – Wagener – Barker classification of the retinal changes in hypertension has provided a simple and excellent means for serial evaluation of the hypertensive patient. Increasing severity of hypertension is associated with focal spasm and progressive general narrowing of the arterioles , as well as the appearance of hemorrhages, exudates, and papilledema. These retinal lesions often produce scotomata, blurred vision and even blindness especially in the presence of papilledema or hemorrhages of the macular area. Hypertensive lesions may develop acutely and if therapy results in significant reduction of blood pressure, may show rapid resolution. Rarely, these lesions resolve without therapy. In contrast, retinal arteriolosclerosis results from endothelial and muscular proliferation, and it accurately reflects similar changes in other organs. Sclerotic changes do not develop as rapidly as hypertensive lesions, nor do they regress appreciably with therapy. As a consequence of increased wall thickness and rigidity, sclerotic arterioles distort and compress the veins as they cross within their common fibrous sheath, and the reflected light streak from the arterioles is changed by the increased opacity of the vessel wall.

Central nervous system dysfunction also occurs frequently in patients with hypertension. Occipital headaches . most often in the morning, are among the most prominent early symptoms of hypertension. Dizziness, light – headedness, vertigo, tinnitus, and dimmed vision or syncope may also be observed, but the more serious manifestations are due to vascular occlusion or hemorrhage.

Renal Effects   Arteriolosclerotic lesions of the afferent
and efferent arterioles and the glomerular capillary tufts are
the most common renal vascular lesions in hypertension and
result in decreased glomerular filtration rate and tubular dysfunction. Proteinuria and microscopic hematuria occur because of glomerular lesions , and approximately 10 percent of
the deaths secondary to hypertension result from renal failure, Blood loss in hypertension occurs not only from renal lesions; epistaxis, hemoptysis, and metrorrhagia also occur
most frequently in these patients.

In general, traditional Chinese treatment of hypertension lowers the blood pressure less but relieves hypertensive
symptoms better than western medicines. Therefore, combined traditional Chinese medicine and western medicine is a
logical approach for hypertension.

Main Points of Pathogenesis

Hypertension is included in the categories of "xuanyun"
(vertigo) and "tou tong"(headache). It is common thought
that hypertension occurs when incoordination between yin
and yang is caused by impairment of seven modes of emotion, improper diet, internal damage and deficiency. The
main injured viscera are heart, liver and kidney.

1. Hyperactivity of liver - yang   It is usually postulated
that long - term emotional, upsets or grief easily lead to

stagnation of the liver – energy with formation of evil fire, manifesting as headache, dizziness, tinnitus, restlessness, flushed face and others. Overexertion or body debility and general hypofunction may induce consumption of blood or deficiency of yin and gradually leads to the inequality of yin and yang in which the yin is unable to inhibit yang – energy and over – activity of yang ensues, and in turn , the hyperactivity of yang may further consumes the yin – fluid which further results in development of liver yang hyperactivity due to deficiency of yin – fluid. Sthenia of liver – yang usually occurs in mild hypertension.

2. Deficiency of the liver – yin and kidney – yin   Liver and kidney is said to come from the same origin. Between them there are the mutual supply of nutrients and the close relationship. Liver stores blood and kidney stores essence. The blood and essence are able to transform each other. Insufficiency of kidney – yin usually causes insufficiency of liver – yin and vice versa, which would lead to the deficiency of the liver – yin and kidney – yin. It usually presents in some of patients with hypertension and probably accounts for the hypertension in these patients.

3. Deficiency of yin leading to hyperactivity of yang   It is a morbid condition due to the consumption of essence, blood and body fluid, which can lead to the inequality of yin and yang , in which the yin is unable to inhibit yang – energy and over – activity of yang ensues, and, in turn, the hyper-

activity of yang may further consumes the yin – fluid. In clinic, the diagnosis may be established by concomitant appearance of the deficiency of liver – yin and kidney – yin accompanying with sthenia of liver – yang.

4. Deficiency of heart – yin　Heart – yin is the nutritious fluid of the heart and a component of blood. It has a close relation to the heart – blood physiologically and pathologically, and also to the condition of lung – yin and kidney – yin. Deficiency of kidney – yin may cause that water fails to inhibit fire which will gradually lead to an excess of fire and eventually result in the deficiency of heart – yin. The common features, such as palpitation, insomnia, dreaminess and amnesia, are sought in most of the patients with hypertension.

5. Deficiency of both yin and yang　It is a morbid condition characterized by simultaneously occurrence of deficiency of yin and yang and usually seen in the later stage of hypertension. The cause is that yang is involved by deficient yin such as kidney damage resulting in chronic renal failure. This type is less than another types in hypertension patients.

6. Deficiency of both vital energy and yin　It is a morbid condition of damage of both yin fluid and yang energy occurring in the course of hypertension in moderate depth. Vital energy is the functions of various organs and tissues of the body, which is included in the categories of yang in traditional Chinese medicine. Deficiency of vita energy may cause

hypofunction of viscera and lowering of metabolism due to insufficiency of yang – energy with failure to warm and nourish
the viscera, manifesting as pale complexion, dizziness, tinnitus, palpitation, shortness of breath, lassitude and spontaneous sweating. deficiency of yin may cause hyperactivity of
fire, manifesting as hot feeling of the palms and soles, red
lips , dry mouth, oliguria with yellowish urine, constipation,
red tongue with no coating, headache and others. In an individual patient when there are simultaneously some of the
symptoms of both efficiency of vital energy and deficiency of
yin, the diagnosis of this type may be established by carefully
examination.

7. Maladjustment of chong and ren channels   It may
result from impairment of the liver and kidney, elderly and
climacteric irregular menstruation and is usually seen in the
female patients with hypertension. Irregular menstruation
usually occurs preceding the amenorrhea. In the menstrual
period , there are obviously fluctuation of the blood pressure
and general malaise, which easily induce to elevate the level
of the blood pressure.

Differential Diagnosis and Treatment

1) Upward exacerbation of liver *yang*

The patients may suffer from pain and distension of
head, vertigo, flushed face, restlessness, insomnia and

numbness of fingers or half side of body. The tongue proper is red in color with yellow coating and the pulse is wiry and rapid.

Therapeutic principle   To suppress hyperactivity of liver and control exacerbation of *yang*.

Principal acupoints   **Gāndiǎn, Wàiláogōng (EX – UE8)**

Supplemental acupoints   **Hégǔ(LI4), Láogōng(PC8), Xīndiǎn** and **Shèndiǎn**. The reducing method is applied to **Gāndiǎn** and **Wàiláogōng(EX – UE8)**; the balanced reinforce – reducing method is applied to **Láogōng (PC8), Xīndiǎn** and **Shèndiǎn**.

2) Upward disturbance of phlegm and turbid fluid

The patients may suffer from vertigo, distension of head, fullness of chest and upper abdomen, vomiting and spitting phlegm and saliva, poor appetite, palpitation of heart, insomnia, heaviness and numbness of limbs. The tongue coating is white and greasy and the pulse is wiry and rolling.

Therapeutic principle   To resolve phlegm, release stasis of collaterals and suppress hyperactivity of liver.

Principal acupoints   **Wàngǔ(SI4)** and **Nèiguān(PC6)**.

Supplemental acupoints   **Yèmén (SJ2), Hòuxī (SI3), Pídiǎn** and **Láogōng(PC8)**.

3) Excessiveness of liver *fire*

The patients may suffer from headache, vertigo, distension of eyes, flushed face and eyes, bitter taste in mouth, dryness in throat, high irritability and angry, constipation and dark urine. The tongue proper is red in color with yellow coating and the pulse is wiry and rapid.

Therapeutic principle　　To clear liver *fire* and control exacerbation of *yang*.

Principal acupoints　　**Gāndiǎn** and **Bāxié(EX − UE9)**.

Supplemental acupoints　　**Yèmén (SJ2)**, **Zhōngzhǔ (SJ3)**, **Yángchí(SJ4)**, **Gāndiǎn** and **Láogōng(PC8)**.

4) Deficiency of liver and kidney *yin*

The patients may suffer from dizziness, vertigo, tinnitus, hotness in heart, palms and soles, dryness in eyes and mouth, night sweating, numbness of limbs, twitching of muscles and insomnia. The tongue proper is red in color with scanty coating and the pulse is thready and rapid or wiry and thready.

Therapeutic principle　　To tonify liver and kidney.

Principal acupoints　　**Nèiguān(PC6)** and **Gāndiǎn**.

Supplemental acupoints　　**Hégǔ (LI4)**, **Yīnxī (HT6)**, **Yángchí(SJ4)**, **Shàoshāng(LU11)** and **Láogōng(PC8)**.

5) Failure of communication between heart and kidney

The patients may suffer from dizziness, tinnitus, soreness and weakness of waist and knee, poor memory, annoyance, palpitation of heart, insomnia and dark urine. The tongue proper is red in color with scanty coating and the pulse is wiry and thready.

Therapeutic principle   To reduce *fire* and enrich water and to communicate heart and kidney.

Principal acupoints   **Nèiguān(PC6)**.

Supplemental acupoints   **Gāndiǎn, Tàiyuān (LU9), Shénmén(HT7), Xīndiǎn** and **Shèndiǎn**.

6) Deficiency of kidney *yang*

The patients may suffer from soreness and weakness of waist and knee, dizziness, tinnitus, mental and physical tiredness, cold body and limbs, frequent night urination, impotence, emission of semen and frequent tremor. The tongue proper is pale and puffy with white coating and the pulse is deep, slow and weak.

Therapeutic principle   To warm *yang* and tonify kidney.

Principal acupoints   **Láogōng(PC8) Nèiguān(PC6)**.

Supplemental acupoints   **Yújì (LU10), Tàiyuān (LU9), Xīndiǎn, Shèndiǎn** and **Yángchí(SJ4)**.

Headache

Headache is a kind of clinically common — subjective symptom. It can be accompanied by various kinds of acute and chronic diseases. This section will mainly discuss some symptoms characterized mainly by headache.

Etiology and Pathogenesis

Yang qi from all meridians may converge to the head and the essence stored in all internal organs may be assembled to supply nutrients to the head. The head is a clean and peaceful organ and it can only receive the clear *qi*, but it can not tolerate the invasion of pathogenic *qi*, which may block the orifices of sense organs to cause headache. The headache may be caused by the following pathological disturbances: deficiency of *qi* and blood and malnutrition of meridians; deficiency of kidney water (*yin*) and exacerbation of liver *yang* to attack the head; stagnation of liver *qi* to produce *fire* pathogen; blockage of circulation of *qi* by stagnated blood or phlegm and turbid fluid; and invasion of external 6 pathogens to block *qi* in meridians, disturb the function of brain and obstruct the orifices of sense organs.

Clinical Manifestations

1. Headache due to Exopathy

1) Headache due to Pathogenic Wind – Cold Pathogen: frequent headache, pain extending to the nape and back, aversion to cold and wind, joy for head – binding, no thirst, thin and whitish tongue fur, floating and tense pulse.

2) Headache due to Pathogenic Wind – Heat: distension and pain in the head, fever, aversion to wind, thirst with desire to drink, dark urine, reddened tongue with thin and yellow fur, floating and rapid pulse.

3) Headache due to Pathogenic Summer – Heat and Dampness: strong binding pain in the head, lassitude of limbs, poor appetite, fullness in the epigastric region, fever, sweating, dysphoria, thirst, greasy fur and slippery pulse.

2. Headache due to Internal Injury

1) Headache due to Abnormal Ascending of Liver – Yang: headache with intermittent dizziness, dysphoria, irritability, insomnia, bitter taste, reddened tongue with thin and yellow fur, taut and forceful pulse.

2) Headache due to Stagnation of Phlegm: Headache with dizziness, fullness in the epigastric region, vomiting, abundant expectoration, whitish and greasy fur, slippery or taut and slippery pulse.

3) Headache due to Deficiency of Blood: Headache and dizziness which become intense with slight labor, weakness, dysphoria, palpitation, shortness of breath, pale complexion, pale tongue with thin and whitish fur, thready and feeble pulse.

4) Headache due to Deficiency of Kidney: Headache with a sensation of emptiness inside the head, dizziness, weakness and lassitude in the loin and legs, emission, leukorrhagia, tinnitus, insomnia, reddened tongue with little fur, thready and feeble pulse.

Differential Diagnosis

1. Headache due to invasion of pathogenic wind into the channels and collaterals: Headache occurs often, especially on exposure to wind. The pain may extend to the nape of the neck and back regions. Thin and white tongue coating, floating pulse.

2. Headache due to upsurge of liver − yang: headache, distension of the head, irritability, hot temper, dizziness, blurring of vision, red tongue with thin and yellow coating, taut and rapid pulse.

3. Headache due to deficiency of both qi and blood: Lingering headache, dizziness, blurring of vision, lassitude, lusterless face, pale tongue with thin and white coating, thin and weak pulse.

1. Body Acupuncture

Principal points　　**Bǎihuì**, **Tàiyáng** (EX – HN5) and **Hégǔ**(LI4)

Supplementary Points　　In the treatment of headache due to invasion of pathogenic wind into channels and collaterals, supplementary points should be selected according to the channel and collateral in which the pain is located. For frontal headache, **Yìntáng**(EX – HN3), **Shàngxīng**(DU23) and **Nèitíng**(ST44); for temporal headache, **Wàiguān**(SJ5) and **Zúlínqì** (GB41); for parietal headache, **Hòuxī** (SI3), **Tàichōng**(LR3) and **Zhìyīn**(BL67); for occipital headache, **Fēngchí**(GB20) and **Kūnlún** (BL60). In the treatment of headache due to upsurge of liver – yang, **Fēngchí** (GB20), **Xiáxī**(GB43) and **Xíngjiān**(LR2) are added. In the treatment of headache due to deficiency of both qi and blood, **Qìhǎi**(RN6), **Zúsānlǐ**(ST36), **Píshū** (BL20) and **Shènshū** (BL23) are added.

Method　　Use the filiform needles to puncture the points with reinforcing method and moxibustion, for headache due to deficiency of both qi and blood, and with the reducing method or even movement for the other two types of headache.

2. Hand Acupuncture

1) Invasion of external pathogens

The patients may suffer from paroxysmal attacks of headache with fixed location and fever. The tongue coating is thin and white in color and the pulse is floating.

Therapeutic principle   To expel wind pathogen and relieve the symptoms of exterior syndrome.

Principal acupoints   **Hòutóudiǎn, Qiántóudiǎn, Piāntóudiǎn** and **Tóudǐngdiǎn**.

Supplemental acupoints   The same as those applied in body acupuncture.

2) Upward attack of exacerbated liver *yang*

The patients may suffer from headache with vertigo, distension of eyes, high irritability and angry, unstable sleeping, annoyance, flushed face, bitter taste in mouth and pain in flank and costal region. The tongue is red in color with yellow coating and the pulse is wiry.

Therapeutical principle   To enrich *yin* and suppress *yang*.

Principal acupoints   **Tàichōng (LR3), Tàixī (KI3)**, and **Tóudǐngdiǎn**.

Supplemental acupoints   **Gāndiǎn, Shèndiǎn, Láogōng (PC8)**.

3) Traumatic headache

The headache is fixed in location and spread all over the head. The tongue proper is dark in color with petechiae and

:he pulse is uneven or wiry and thready.

Therapeutic principle   To promote blood circulation and
:elease stasis in collaterals.

Principal acupoints   **Hégǔ(LI4)** and **Hòuxī(SI3)**.

Supplemental acupoints   **Shàoshāng(LU11), Pídiǎn**.

Common Cold

Common cold is one of the most common diseases, and is characterized by fever, aversion to cold, nasal obstruction, runny nose, sneezing, coughing and headache. This disease can occur in all four seasons, but more commonly in winter and spring when there is a drastic change in weather, and in cases of all ages. The younger the patients are, the more the complications there will be. This is the principal characteristic of the common cold of children, which does not appear in adults.

Etiology and Pathogenesis

Pathogenic wind is the predominant etiological factor in colds. It invades the upper respiratory tract and the body surface when body resistance is low, which typically occurs when there is a sudden climatic change. The pathogenic

wind combines with cold in winter, heat in spring and damp
– heat in summer, taking advantage of untimely climatic
changes to attack the body.

The attack on the body is closely related to body resistance, so if one's vital energy is low due to an irregular life
style, drenching by rain, negligence regarding changes in
temperature or overfatigue, the likelihood of invasion increases. A patient with chronic bronchitis or bronchiectasis is
also vulnerable. Furthermore, the body's constitution plays
a role in the affection. A person with a yang deficiency is
susceptible to wind – cold, and one with a yin deficiency is
susceptible to wind – heat.

Because pathogenic wind invades through the upper respiratory tract and the body surface, pathological changes are
confined to these portions of the body. When pathogenic factors obstruct the upper respiratory tract, respiratory symptoms occur, such as cough and stuffy nose. The confronta-
tion between the body's resistance and pathogenic factors at
the superficial portion of the body results in chilliness and
fever.

In case of Delicate visceral organs, thin skin and weak
Wei – system in combination with sudden change of the
weather, the six exopathogenic factors are apt to attack the
superficies to cause failure of superficial qi, disorder of opening and closing function of skin striae and inhibition of yang
energy, manifested by fever and chills, headache, running

and stuffy nose, cough etc.

In young cases of common cold, fever may be severe. It is because young children are of pure yang bodies and the invasion of evils is liable to bring about heat. Because of the delicate lungs in young cases, when they are attacked by evils, the lung – qi will stagnate, and qi will be out of order, and the body fluids may accumulate to form sputum, obstructing the air passages, causing productive cough. The spleen of young cases is not fully developed. If their diet is not proper after being attacked, the digestive function may be involved, milk and food may stagnate in the middle – jiao. They may present with distention of gastric cavity and abdomen, poor appetite for milk and food, vomiting or diarrhea, and some other dyspeptic symptoms. The invasion of evils will cause heat and fire, affecting the spirit, leading to vigilance and restlessness, even infantile convulsion. This is known as cold with convulsion in pediatrics.

Main Points of Diagnosis

1. Main Symptoms and Signs: It is mostly manifested by sudden onset, fever with no or little sweat, running and stuffy nose, sore throat, mild cough, etc. The body temperature is varied with different strains of pathogen type of disease and individual condition. Infants and younger children tend to have higher temperature than the older ones, some-

times reaching 40℃, but with better general condition. Older children have more severe localized symptoms of the nose, pharynx and throat.

2. **Complications**: In infants and young children, it is usually associated with high fever, convulsion or vomiting, diarrhea, abdominal pain, anorexia or productive cough, and even bronchitis or pneumonia.

3. Some acute infectious diseases such as measles, chicken pox, scarlet fever, epidemic mumps, epidemic encephalomyelitis, etc. have the same manifestations as colds in their early stages, but different features will soon be found later. So early identification is very necessary.

Differential Diagnosis and Treatment

1) Wind cold type of common cold

The patients may suffer from headache, fever, chillness, sore pain of body, nasal obstruction, running nose, sneezing, cough, no thirst and no sweating. The tongue proper is pale with white thin coating and the pulse is floating or floating and tense.

Therapeutic principle   To expel cold pathogen from body surface and to disperse *qi* of lungs and control cough.

Principal acupoints   **Shāngyáng (LI1)**, **Shàoshāng (LU11) and Hòutóudiǎn**.

Supplemental acupoints   **Yújì (LU10)**, **Yíngxiāng**

(LI20), **Fèidiǎn** and **Yānhóudiǎn**.

The moxibustion with ginger is applied to **Fèidiǎn** and **Yíngxiāng**(LI20) with moxa cones changed for 5 times; pricking therapy is applied on the points **Shàoshāng**(LU11) and **Shāngyáng**(LI1); and the decoction of *Rhizoma Zingiberis Recens* 25 g, *Bulbus Allii Fistulosi* 15 g and *Folium Perillae* 15 g may be orally administered. 2) Wind heat type of common cold

The patients may suffer from headache, high fever, mild chillness, soreness and distending discomfort of joints all over the body, slight sweating, cough with yellow sputum, nasal obstruction and running nose. The tongue proper is red in color with yellow thin coating and the pulse is floating and rapid.

Therapeutic principle   To disperse *qi* of lungs, expel pathogen from body surface, clear heat and resolve phlegm.

Principal acupoints   **Hégǔ**(LI4), **Fèidiǎn** and **Qūchí** (**LI11**).

Supplemental acupoints   **Yānhóudiǎn**, **Yújì** (LU10), **Yángchí**(SJ4).

The reducing technique is applied to **Hégǔ** (LI4), **Fèidiǎn** and **Yújì**(LU10).

3) Dampness type of common cold

The patients may suffer from heaviness and distension of head, low fever and chillness, soreness, heaviness and pain of joints, cough with dull sound and white sticky sputum, fullness of chest and upper abdomen, poor appetite and incomplete bowel movement. The tongue coating is white greasy or yellow greasy and the pulse is soft and moderate.

Therapeutic principle   To eliminate dampness from body surface, release stasis in spleen and stomach and resolve turbid fluid.

Principal acupoints   **Yújì(LU10)** and **Fèidiǎn**.

Supplemental acupoints   **Bāxié (EX – UE9), Sānjiāodiǎn, Láogōng(PC8), Pídiǎn**.

The moxibustion with atractylodes is applied at **Sānjiāodiǎn** with moxa cones in a size of a wheat grain and changed for 5 times; the bleeding therapy is applied at **Yújì (LU10)**; and the patent herbal drug, Huoxiang Zhengqi Pills may be orally administered, 9 g tid.

4) Summer – heat type of common cold

The patients may suffer from headache, annoyance, fever, thirst, slight chillness, cough, chest distress, poor appetite and short stream of dark urine. The tongue proper is red in color with yellow thin coating and the pulse is rapid.

Therapeutic principle   To clear summer – heat from body surface, resolve dampness and regulate spleen and stomach.

Principal acupoint   **Bāxié(EX – UE9)**.

Supplemental acupoints   **Shāngyáng(LI1), Shàoshāng (LU11), Yújì(LU10), Sānjiāodiǎn, Pídiǎn**.

The bleeding therapy is applied to **Bāxié(EX – UE9)**,

Shàoshāng(LU11) and Shāngyáng(LI1); the reducing technique is applied to Yújì(LU10); and the balanced reinforce –
reducing technique is applied to all other acupoints. The decoction of fresh lotus leaf 20 g, skin of watermelon 50 g,
peel of mung bean 20 g, flower of white lablab seed 15 g and
Bohe (field mint) 10 g is drunk as tea.

Influenza

Influenza, an infectious disease of respiratory tract, is caused by influenza viruses. The disease has extremely strong infectivity, transmitted by means of droplets. People are very susceptible to influenza and sometimes pandemics may happen over the world. Although influenza may occur at all seasons, it tends to appear during winter and spring. This disease, in traditional Chinese medicine is called *Shixing ganmao*.

Main Points of Diagnosis

1. A large number of patients are affected within a short period with clinical features of fever, headache and myalgia.

2. Clinical features

1) The onset of the disease is abrupt, with marked general toxemic symptoms such as chill, fever, headache, myal-

gia, weakness, etc.

2) Symptoms referable to the respiratory tract such as stuffy nose, rhinorrhea, sore throat and dry cough are usually mild. In some cases, symptoms of the digestive tract such as loss of appetite, nausea, vomiting, abdominal pain and diarrhea may be present.

3) High fever, chest pain, cough, bloody sputum, dyspnea and even coma may occur in severe cases.

4) Physical examination reveals acutely ill complexion and malar flush with congestion of conjunctival and nasopharyngeal mucosa. In patients with influenzal pneumonia or secondary bacterial pneumonia, the respiratory sounds are diminished. Diffuse moist rales may be heard over the lung fields.

3. Laboratory test show a decreased leukocyte count and the ratio of neutrophils to leukocytes, while the lymphocytes count may be relatively elevated. Mucosal imprint from inferior nasal conchae may show inclusions of influenza virus. This is valuable for the early diagnosis. In serological examinations, hemagglutination inhibition test or complement fixation test can be used for the diagnosis. Viral isolation is helpful in confirming the type of pathogen.

Differential Diagnosis and Treatment

1. Wind – cold Syndrome

Main Symptoms and Signs: Severe aversion to cold, slight fever, absence of sweat, headache, aching pain of extremities, stuffy nose with nasal discharge, cough with thin sputum, thin and whitish coating of tongue, floating and tight pulse.

Therapeutic Principles: Relieving exterior syndrome with the drugs pungent in flavor and warm in property, ventilating the lung and expelling pathogenic cold.

2. Wind – heat Syndrome

Main Symptoms and Signs: High fever, slight aversion to cold, headache, sore throat with congestion, expectoration of yellowish sputum, thirst or even epistaxis, reddened tongue with thin and yellowish fur, floating and rapid pulse.

Therapeutic Principles: Relieving exterior syndrome with the drugs pungent in flavor and cool in property, promoting the dispersing function of the lung and clearing up pathogenic heat. The treatment are similar to those given for **Common Cold**.

Cough

Cough is one of the most frequently seen respiratory symptoms, which occurs in all four seasons, especially in winter and spring. The incidence is high in babies under three years of age. The younger the cases are, the more severe the pathological conditions will be. Cough is often caused by invasion of external pathogenic factors, its duration short and its prognosis good.

When lung and defensive qi are weak, the external pathogenic wind－cold or wind－heat is likely to invade the lung system via the mouth, nose and skin pores, thus impairing the function of the lung in dispersing and descending. Subsequently, cough will result. Retention of phlegm－damp in the spleen and lung can also cause cough when induced by invasion of external pathogenic factors.

Etiology and Pathogenesis

1. Cough attacked by exogenous pathogenic factors.

When weather is changeable in winter and spring, six exogenous pathogenic factors will easily attack the lung, resulting in cough due to impairment of purifying and descending function of the lung and abnormal rising of lung – qi. As the result of the sluggishness of lung – qi, the interior retention and accumulation of the body fluid will form sputum, obstructing the air passage and inducing productive cough.

2. Stagnation of phlegm in the interior

The stagnation of dampness may be transformed into sputum which will store in the lung, block the air passage and inhibit ventilation.

3. Weak constitution

People are apt to be invaded by exogenous pathogenic factors if they are congenitally deficient and weak in constitution. The invasion brings about recurrent cough. Chronic cough will injure the spleen and the lung and result in cough by the internal injury due to deficiency of both the spleen and the lung, and the consumption of the lung – yin.

Main Points of Diagnosis

1. The initial onset of the cough caused by exogenous pathogenic factors is mostly accompanied by cold symptoms such as chilliness, fever, stuffy nose with watery discharge, headache, general muscular pains, redness and itching of the throat. After one or two days, it is chiefly marked by cough. At first, the cough may present with deep, loud or raucous sound, which is mild during the day and severe at night, associated with vomiting, and thin whitish or thick yellowish sputum. However, young children are unable to spit.

2. Cough caused by internal injury is commonly seen in the cases with delicate constitution and malnutrition. These people are likely to catch a cold and will be more severely attacked by pathogenic factors. The course of the disease is rather long, manifested by cough low cough with thin whitish or less thick sputum or associated with fever.

Differential Diagnosis and Treatment

1) Cough due to external pathogens

(1) Cough due to wind cold pathogen

The patients may suffer from cough with thin sputum, nasal obstruction and running nose, itching in the throat, hoarseness of voice, or fever and chillness, headache, pain of body without sweating. The tongue coating is thin and white and the pulse is floating and tense.

Therapeutic principle　To disperse *qi* of lungs, expel cold pathogen and stop cough.

Principal acupoints　**Fèidiǎn** and **Pídiǎn**.

Supplemental acupoints　**Yújì(LU10)**, **Yángchí(SJ4)**.

(2) Cough due to wind heat pathogen

The patients may suffer from cough with yellow sticky sputum, dryness in mouth, sore throat, or fever, chillness induced by blowing wind and spontaneous sweating. The tongue coating is thin and yellow and the pulse is floating and rapid.

Therapeutic principle　To disperse *qi* of lungs, expel pathogens from body surface and clear heat.

Principal acupoints　**Fèidiǎn** and **Kéchuǎndiǎn**.

Supplemental acupoints　**Hòuxī (SI3)** and **Yángchí (SJ4)**.

Tàiyuān(LU9), **Hégǔ(LI4)** and **Fèishū(BL13)** may be used to treat patients with dry cough but without sputum, caused by injury of lungs by dry heat.

2) Cough due to injury of lungs by liver *fire*

The patients may suffer from cough, shortness of breath, pain radiated to both flanks, dryness in throat and fluched face. The tongue proper is red in color with yellow coating and the pulse is wiry and rapid.

Therapeutic principle   To suppress hyperactivity of liver and clear lung heat.

Principal acupoints   **Hégǔ (LI4)**, **Fèidiǎn** and **Shèndiǎn**.

Supplemental acupoints   **Gāndiǎn, Tàiyuān(LU9)** and **Yānhóudiǎn**.

Bronchial Asthma

Bronchial asthma is an allergic respiratory disease with recurrent attacks. Patients with asthma usually have a history of exudative conditions such as eczema, urticaria and angioneurotic edema. It is more commonly seen in children of four or five. Once they are exposed to allergens like bacterial or viral infection, flower powder, mites and dust, or after they take in fish, shrimps and protein, asthmatic attacks may occur. It may be often induced by sudden changes of the weather, overwork and mental irritation. Asthma is more common in spring and autumn, being prone to occur repeatedly. In infants and young children, it appears mostly like asthmatic bronchitis. With the growth of the children the frequency of attacks gradually reduces and the disease is even relieved. But when they grow older, the disease will recur. It is difficult to cure completely, usually becoming a life − long disorder.

Etiology and Pathogenesis

Bronchial asthma results when exopathic factors act on the endopathic factors. The patient is generally weak in constitution and deficient in the functions of the lung, spleen and kidney. The deficiency of the lung may result in retention of water, the dysfunction of the spleen in water transportation, and deficiency of kidney in activating qi to promote diuresis. Retention and accumulation of water and dampness form turbid sputum, which stores in the interior. As a result, the sick child usually manifested by exudative conditions, showing pale complexion, fatness, recurrent eczema, loose muscle, and rumbling sound of the sputum in the throat, etc. .

Because of the deficiency of lung − energy, the **yang** of the defensive function fails to strengthen the striae, which in turn makes one subject to attacks of exogenous pathogenic factors. In this case, if there are sudden changes of weather, the invasion of exopathogens into the body, the exposure to some substances, such as flower powder, mites, parasites and dust, irregular diet, over − eating of uncooked, cold, salty and acid food or taking in fish, shrimps and protein, the latent phlegm will be irritated, obstructing the air passage, making lung − qi unable to go up and down, therefore causing sudden attacks of asthma. Asthma that is due to retention of cold − type phlegm in the interior caused by the attack of wind – cold evil, internal injury by improper diet or deficiency of **yang** is known as cold – type asthma. Asthma that is due to deficiency of **yin** , accumulation of phlegm – heat in the lung or the transformation of cold – type phlegm into heat is known as heat – type asthma. If recurrent attacks of asthma further injure the vital essence of the lung, spleen and the kidney, the disease may present as deficient – type asthma with shortness of breath, bronchial wheezing when moving, and productive cough, which are commonly seen at the remission stage of the disease. Because the disease is caused by deficiency in origin and excess in superficiality, or a deficiency syndrome complicated with excess, it is difficult to be completely cured. When weather suddenly changes, diet is improper, and the mental irritated, the combination of exopathogens and endopathogens leads to recurrent attacks of asthma.

Main Points of Diagnosis

Bronchial asthma is divided into two different stages: attack and remission.

1. Typical Attack: It is marked by sudden onset or by the presymptoms of stuffy nose, sneezing, itching in the throat and oppressed feeling in the chest followed by asthma, shortness of breath, dyspnea, sound of sputum in thethroat, restlessness, failure of horizontal position, pale complexion,

cyanosis of the lips and fingers, and cold sweat on the fore-head. At beginning, there is dry cough, and later, the amount of sputum gradually increases. Once the sputum is removed, the attack will be relieved. The duration of the attack varies from a few minutes to several hours. A few children are found in status asthmaticus.

2. **Signs:** Stethoscope examination finds obvious diminution of respiration in the two lungs, prolonged expiratory phase and wheezing all over the two lungs. In chronic patients, drumstick finger and barrel chest are commonly seen.

3. **X－ray Examination:** X－ray examination of the chest reveals changes of emphysema. When secondary infection occurs, patchy shadows can be observed.

4. **Laboratory Test:** White cell count and neutrophilic granulocytes are generally normal; eosinophilic granulocytes increase by more than 5%; when secondary infection presents, white cell count and neutrophilic granulocytes may increase.

Differential Diagnosis and Treatment

1) Attack of wind and cold pathogens to body surface

The patients may suffer from asthma, chest fullness, profuse clear and thin sputum, headache, chillness, or fever, but no thirst. The tongue coating is white, slippery and greasy and the pulse is floating and rolling.

Therapeutic principle   To disperse qi of lungs, expel cold pathogen from body surface and control asthma.

Principal acupoints   **Fèidiǎn, Pídiǎn** and **Shèndiǎn**.

Supplemental acupoints   **Hégǔ(LI4)**, **Hòuxī(SI3)** and **Bāxié(EX - UE9)**.

The moxibustion with ginger is applied to **Fèidiǎn** with moxa cones in a size of a wheat grain and changed for 3 times; and the warm acupuncture is applied to **Shèndiǎn** and **Hòuxī(SI3)**.

2) Obstruction of heat and phlegm in lungs

The patients may suffer from asthma, rough breath, frequent fever with annoyance, profuse yellow and sticky sputum and chest pain induced by cough. The tongue proper is red in color with yellow coating and the pulse is rapid.

Therapeutic principle   To clear heat in lungs and resolve phlegm.

Principal acupoints   **Fèidiǎn** and **Xiàochuǎndiǎn**.

Supplemental acupoints   **Gōngsūn(SP4)**.

3) **Deficiency of lung and kidney** qi

The patients may suffer from asthma, shortness of breath with long expiration and short inspiration and worse after physical exertion, weakness, pale complexion, restlessness, hotness in heart, palms and soles and cold leg. The tongue proper is pale with thin and white coating and the pulse is thready and faint.

Therapeutic principle   To tonify kidney and lung *qi* .

Principal acupoints   **Tàiyuān(LU9)** and **Fèidiǎn**.

Supplemental acupoints   **Fèishū(BL13)** and **Shèndiǎn**.

The moxibustion with aconite is applied at **Fèishū(BL13)** and **Shèndiǎn**.

Hiccup

Hiccup is a symptom with repeated short hiccup noise in throat produced by quick squeeze of air out of the throat.

Etiology and Pathogenesis

The hiccup is usually caused by the intake of cold or spicy food or the administration of drugs with cold nature. The emotional disturbance, such as angry and depression may stir up the liver *qi* to attack the lungs and stomach and irritate the contraction of diaphragm to push the stomach *qi* with phlegm rushing upward. In chronic patients with deficiency of spleen and kidney *yang*, the downward transporting function of stomach may be impaired and the promoting inspiration function of kidney may be also impaired. Therefore, the stomach *qi* may be pushed upward by the contraction of diaphragm to cause hiccup.

Differential Diagnosis and Treatment

1) Excessive type

(1) Upward flaming of stomach *fire*

The hiccup noise is loud and the air is suddenly discharged. The patients may also suffer from foul smell from mouth, annoyance and fullness, preference to drink cold water, short stream of dark urine and constipation. The tongue proper is red in color with yellow coating and the pulse is rolling and rapid.

Therapeutic principle   To clear heat and suppress upward rushing of stomach *qi*.

Principal acupoint   **Pídiǎn, Nèiguān(PC6)**.

Supplemental acupoints   **Hégǔ (LI4)** and **Shàoshāng (LU11)**.

(2) Cold pathogen in stomach

The hiccup noise is low and the air is slowly discharged. The hiccup may be reduced and relieved by treatment of hotness and it may be worse by treatment of coldness. The appetite of the patients is poor. The tongue proper is pale with thin and white coating and the pulse is slow and moderate or deep and moderate.

Therapeutic principle   To warm spleen and stomach, expel cold pathogen and stop hiccup.

Principal acupoint   **Pídiǎn**.

Supplemental acupoints   **Zúsānlǐ (ST36)**. The moxibustion with ginger is applied to **Zúsānlǐ(ST36)** with moxa cones in a size of a wheat grain and changed for 5 times until the local skin is flushed; and the warm acupuncture is applied at **Pídiǎn** for 5 minutes.

2) Deficient type

(1) Deficiency of spleen and stomach *yang*

The hiccup noise is low and feeble. The patients may suffer from weakness and no desire to speak, pale complexion, cold hands and feet and sensitiveness of upper abdomen to coldness. The tongue proper is pale with thin and white coating and the pulse is moderate and weak.

Therapeutic principle　To warm and tonify spleen and stomach.

Principal acupoint　**Pídiǎn**.

Supplemental acupoints　**Sānjiāodiǎn, Gōngsūn(SP4)** and **Nèiguān(PC6)**.

(2) Insufficiency of stomach *yin*

The hiccup noise is quick and continuous and the patients also suffer from annoyance and dryness in mouth and tongue. The tongue proper is dry and red in color and the pulse is thready and rapid.

Therapeutic principle　To tonify stomach *yin* and stop hiccup.

Principal acupoints　**Zúsānlǐ(ST36)** and **Pídiǎn**.

Supplemental acupoints　**Shàoshāng (LU11), Zhōngzhǔ(SJ3)**.

Stomachache

Stomachache is a common symptom of acute and chronic gastritis, stomach and duodenal peptic ulcer, ptosis of stomach, stomach cancer and some diseases of liver and gallbladder. In patients with stomachache, the pain is located in the upper abdomen between xiphoid process and umbilicus.

Etiology and Pathogenesis

As a reservoir of water and food, the stomach can store and digest food and the normal function of stomach is to downward transport the its contents. The attack of cold pathogen to the stomach may block the meridian and cause spasm and pain of stomach; the worriment and angry may interfere the function to disperse liver qi and the stagnated liver qi may adversely attack the stomach to cause stagnation of stomach qi and pain; the lingering pain of stomach may damage the collaterals and blood vessels to cause hematemesis and tarry stool; the overeating of cold, greasy, sweet and spicy food may cause stagnation of food in stomach with pain due to stagnation of stomach qi.

Differential Diagnosis and Treatment

1) Attack of cold pathogen to stomach

The patients may suffer from spasm and pain of upper abdomen, sensitiveness of upper abdomen to coldness, pale complexion and extremely cold limbs. . The tongue proper is pale with thin and white coating and the pulse is wiry and tense.

Therapeutic principle   To expel cold pathogen, warm stomach, release spasm and stop pain.

Principal acupoints   **Pídiǎn**, **Zúsānlǐ (ST36)** and **Nèiguān(PC6)**.

Supplemental acupoints   **Hégǔ(LI4)**, **Nèitíng(ST44)**, **Yèmén(SJ2)**. The acupuncture followed by moxibustion is applied to **Zúsānlǐ(ST36)** and **Pídiǎn**.

2) Attack of liver qi to stomach

The patients may suffer from distension and pain in upper abdomen and radiation of pain to bilateral flanks, belching, regurgitation of sour fluid and vomiting of bitter fluid. The tongue proper is pale and scattered with tooth prints on its borders, the tongue coating is thin and white in color and the pulse is wiry.

Therapeutic principle   To disperse and adjust liver *qi* and regulate stomach *qi* .

Principal acupoints   **Gōngsūn(SP4)** and **Hégǔ(LI4)**.

Supplemental acupoints   **Sānjiāodiǎn**.

3) Attack of cold pathogen to deficient spleen and stomach

The patients may suffer from dull pain in upper abdomen, regurgitation of clear water, preference warmth to coolness, reduction of pain by palpation, mental and physical tiredness and cool limbs. The tongue coating is white is color and the pulse is moderate and weak.

Therapeutic principle   To adjust and strengthen spleen and stomach.

Principal acupoints   **Pídiǎn** and **Sānjiāodiǎn**.

Supplemental acupoints   **Yújì (LU10)**, **Liángmén (ST21)**.

The moxibustion with aconite or ginger is applied to **Sānjiāodiǎn** with moxa cones in a size of a pit of date and changed for 3 times until the local skin is flushed.

4) Stagnation of food

The patients may suffer from distension and pain of upper abdomen, belching of foul gas and regurgitation of sour fluid, anorexia, constipation or diarrhea. The tongue proper is red in color with yellow and greasy coating and the pulse is wiry and rolling.

Therapeutic principle   To promote digestion and release stagnation of food.

Principal acupoints   **Nèitíng (ST**44) and **Zhōngwǎn** (**RN**12).

Supplemental acupoints   The reducing technique is applied to **Sānjiāodiǎn,** and **Gōngsūn(SP**4).

The mixed powder of notoginseng 5 g, bletilla tuber 9 g and ass－hide glue (melted) 5 g is orally administered with rice soup for patients with stomachache and tarry stool. The patients should be constantly examined to rule out malignant diseases.

Vomiting

Vomiting is a common symptom of stomach with its contents to be reversely casted out of the mouth with or without a vomiting noise. It is called dry vomiting in traditional Chinese medicine, if only the vomiting voice occurs without any vomitus casted out of the mouth.

Etiology and Pathogenesis

The spleen is in charge of digestion and transportation of food. The stomach can receive and digest water and food and the normal function of stomach is to downward transport its contents. If the normal downward transporting function of stomach is disturbed, the vomiting may occur. The pathogenic factors of vomiting can be divided into excessive and deficient types. The stomach heat, stagnation of qi, phlegm and turbid fluid, stagnation of food and adverse attack of liver *qi* to stomach are the excessive pathogenic factors to cause vomiting; but the deficiency of spleen and stomach *yang* in chronic patients with poor function to digest water and food is the deficient pathogenic factor to cause vomiting. The cold pathogen in stomach, deficiency of liver and stomach *yin* and attack of liver wind to stomach are also the pathogenic factors of vomiting.

Differential Diagnosis and Treatment

1) Wind, cold and dampness pathogens

The patients may suffer from prompt vomiting, fever, chillness, pain of head and body, discomfort, fullness or distension of upper abdomen. The tongue proper is pale with white and greasy coating and the pulse is deep and moderate.

Therapeutic principle　To expel pathogens from body surface, resolve turbid fluid and stop vomiting.

Principal acupoints　**Nèiguān(PC6)** and **Pídiǎn**.

Supplemental acupoints　**Sānjiāodiǎn** and **Hégǔ(LI4)**.

The moxibustion with ginger is applied to **Pídiǎn** with moxa cones changed for 5 time; the moxibustion with pepper paste is applied with moxa cones changed for 5 times in patients with violent cold pathogen.

2) Stagnation of food

The patients may suffer from vomiting, fullness and distension of upper abdomen, belching of foul gas and regurgitation of sour fluid and anorexia.

Therapeutic principle   To promote digestion, release stagnation of food, regulate function of stomach and suppress adverse ascending of stomach *qi* .

Principal acupoints   **Zhōngwǎn** (**RN**12) and **Wèichángtòngdiǎn**.

Supplemental acupoints   **Pídiǎn, Hégǔ(LI**4**)** .

3) Stagnation of *qi* of liver and gallbladder

The patients may suffer from distension of chest and upper abdomen, pain of flank and costal region, frequent belching and vomiting of sour and bitter fluid. The border of tongue is red in color with thin and yellow or greasy coating and the pulse is wiry.

Therapeutic principle   To disperse liver *qi*, promote discharge of bile, suppress adverse ascending of stomach *qi* and stop vomiting.

Principal acupoints   **Nèiguān(PC**6**)** and **Sānjiāodiǎn**.

Supplemental acupoints   **Pídiǎn, Gāndiǎn, Gōngsūn (SP**4**)** .

4) Deficiency and weakness of spleen and stomach

The patients may suffer from weakness of limbs, vertigo, vomiting, poor appetite, sallow complexion and loose stool. The tongue proper is pale and the pulse is soft, moderate and weak.

Therapeutic principle   To warm and strengthen spleen and stomach, regulate function of stomach and stop vomiting.

Principal acupoints **Sānjiāodiǎn, Zúsānlǐ**(ST36) and **Gōngsūn**(SP4).

Supplemental acupoints **Pídiǎn**. The moxibustion with atractylodes is applied to **Zúsānlǐ** (ST36) and **Sānjiāodiǎn** with moxa cones changed for 5 times; or the moxibustion with aconite is applied to the same acupoints with moxa cones changed for 3 times until the local skin is flushed.

Ptosis of Stomach

Ptosis of stomach is a disease common in weak and emaciated patients with the stomach in an abnormally low position below the umbilicus.

Etiology and Pathogenesis

The spleen is in charge of digestion and transportation of food and controls limbs and muscles; and the stomach can receive and digest water and food. Therefore, they are the fundamental organs to supply nutrients to nourish all internal organs and external structures of the body after birth. The sinking of spleen qi, weakness of spleen and stomach, deficiency of liver and spleen yin, obstruction of meridians by phlegm and turbid fluid and the intake of improper food are the important pathogenic factors of this disease to cause reduction of tension of stomach, looseness of ligaments of liver and stomach and descent of stomach to an abnormally low position.

Differential Diagnosis and Treatment

1) Deficiency of spleen and stomach *qi*

The patients may suffer from dull pain of upper abdomen, mental tiredness, weakness of limbs, shortness of breath and no desire to speak, sallow complexion, leanness of body, abdominal distension worse after meal and better in lying posture, splashing sound in abdomen, poor appetite, loose stool and long stream of clear urine. The tongue proper is pale with thin and white coating and the pulse is moderate and weak.

Therapeutic principle To tonify *qi* of spleen and stomach and to raise up *yang* of spleen and stomach.

Principal acupoint **Zhōngwǎn(RN12)**.

Supplemental acupoints **Pídiǎn, Sānjiāodiǎn, Zúsānlǐ (ST36)**.

2) Deficiency of liver and spleen *yin*

The patients may suffer from pain in upper abdomen, annoyance, hotness in heart, palms and soles, abdominal distension worse after meal, dull pain in flank and costal region, dryness in mouth, hiccup, belching, insomnia and dreaminess. The tongue proper is red in color with scanty coating and the pulse is wiry and thready.

Therapeutic principle   To tonify *yin* and adjust liver and spleen.

Principal acupoints   **Nèiguān (PC6)** and **Zhōngwǎn (RN12)**.

Supplemental acupoints   **Pídiǎn, Guīlái (ST29), Sānjiāodiǎn**.

3) Blockage of phlegm and dampness

The patients may suffer from pain and distension of upper abdomen, constant nausea, occasional vomiting of saliva and fluid, intestinal gurgling sound, frequent hiccup, belching and poor appetite. The tongue proper is pale with thin and white coating and the pulse is rolling.

Therapeutic principle   To strengthen spleen and stomach, eliminate dampness and resolve phlegm.

Principal acupoints   **Pídiǎn** and **Zhōngwǎn(RN12)**.

Supplemental acupoints   **Zúsānlǐ(ST36), Hégǔ(LI4)**.

4) Stagnation of liver *qi* and deficiency of spleen

The patients may suffer from dizziness, headache, weakness of limbs, pain in bilateral flanks and costing region, insomnia, abdominal distension, poor appetite and alternation of hard and loose stool. The tongue proper is pale with tooth prints on its borders and the pulse is wiry.

Therapeutic principle   To release stagnation of liver *qi* and strengthen spleen.

Principal acupoints   **Nèiguān (PC6)** and **Yángchí (SJ4)**.

Supplemental acupoints **Pídiǎn**.

During the therapeutic period, the patients should be on a diet regimen of semiliquid food with rich nutrients and they should also have enough rest. The clockwise rotating massage on the abdomen may be applied for 30 min twice a day. The physical exercise of upside down on shoulders and back, sit – ups and holding flexed knees may be done to strengthen abdominal muscles.

Abdominal Pain

Abdominal pain is a common symptom of many diseases caused by cold or heat pathogen, stagnation of food, stagnation of qi, deficiency of blood and intestinal parasites.

Etiology and Pathogenesis

The pathogenic factors of abdominal pain can be divided into cold, heat, excessive and deficient types. The external cold pathogen may invade the abdomen and attack Jueyin meridian; the intake of too much cold and uncooked food may injure Yang in body and imperial the digestive function; and the trauma may cause blockage of qi in meridians to produce pain.

Differential Diagnosis and Treatment

1) Excessive syndrome

(1) Abdominal pain caused by cold pathogen

The patients may suffer from acute abdominal colic pain worsened by attack of coldness, no thirst, long stream of clear urine and passage of loose stool. The tongue proper is pale with white and greasy coating and the pulse is deep and tense.

Therapeutic principle   To warm spleen and stomach, expel cold pathogen and stop pain.

Principal acupoints   **Pídiǎn, Hégǔ (LI4)** and **Xiǎochángdiǎn**.

Supplemental acupoints   **Dàchángdiǎn, Sānjiāodiǎn**.

The moxibustion with ginger is applied to **Sānjiāodiǎn** and **Pídiǎn** with moxa cones in a size of a pit of date and changed for 5 times and the warm acupuncture is applied at **Dàchángdiǎn** for 30 minutes.

(2) Abdominal pain caused by heat pathogen

The patients may suffer from abdominal pain sensitive to palpation, abdominal distension and discomfort, severe thirst with desire to drink much water, spontaneous sweating, short stream of dark urine and constipation. The tongue proper is red in color with yellow coating and the pulse is full and rapid or wiry and rapid.

Therapeutic principle   To clear heat by purgation, relieve spasm and stop pain.

Principal acupoints   **Tiānshū(ST25)**, **Xiǎochángdiǎn**.

Supplemental   acupoints   **Nèitíng** (**ST44**), **Dàchángdiǎn**, **Hégǔ(LI4)**.

(3) Abdominal pain caused by stagnation of food

The patients may suffer from anorexia, belching of foul smell and regurgitation of sour fluid, and pain and distension of upper abdomen, intolerable to palpation. The abdominal pain may produce a desire to pass stool and it may be relieved after bowel movement. The tongue proper is red in color with yellow and greasy coating and the pulse is rolling and forceful.

Therapeutic principle   To promote digestion and release stagnation of food.

Principal acupoints   **Dàchángdiǎn** and **Xiǎochángdiǎn**.

Supplemental acupoints   **Pídiǎn**, **Wèichángtòngdiǎn**. The moxibustion with rhubarb is applied to **Dàchángdiǎn** with moxa cones changed for 5 times. (4) Abdominal pain caused by stagnation of qi and blood

The patients may suffer from abdominal pain radiated to lower abdomen or to indefinite directions. The petechiae are spread over the tongue proper and the coating is thin; and the pulse is wiry.

Therapeutic principle   To adjust circulation of qi and

blood.

    Principal acupoints   **Hégǔ(LI4)** and **Dàchángdiǎn**.

    Supplemental   acupoints   **Zúsānlǐ (ST36)**, **Xiǎochángdiǎn**.

    2) Deficient syndrome

The patients may suffer from intermittent dull pain in abdomen, hatred of coldness and preference of hotness and pressure applied to abdomen, shortness of breath and weakness of body. The tongue proper is pale with thin and white coating and the pulse is thready and weak.

    Therapeutic principle   To warm spleen and stomach and tonify qi.

    Principal acupoints   **Mìngméndiǎn** and **Sānjiāodiǎn**.

    Supplemental acupoints   **Pídiǎn, Dàchángdiǎn**.

Diarrhea

Diarrhea is a disease to pass watery or loose stool in increased times per day.

Etiology and Pathogenesis

The diarrhea is a disease more common in summer and autumn seasons and the chief pathogenic organs are Zhongjiao (middle energizer), small intestine and colon. The important pathogenic factors are cold, dampness, summer – heat and heat pathogens and among them the dampness is the chief pathogen to cause diarrhea.

What does "the excessive dampness often causes diarrhea." mean? The overeating or intake of improper food, such as too much greasy and sweet food may cause stagnation of food and damage to spleen and stomach. The external pathogens and stagnation of food can block the spleen Yang.

The digestive function of spleen and stomach, the transporting function of colon and the function to separating clear and turbid body fluid of small intestine may be disturbed by the pathogenic factors mentioned above. The diarrhea is caused by the dysfunction of Zhongjiao to adjust upward and downward transportation of qi and the failure of small intestine to separate clear and turbid fluid. The accumulated liver qi due to emotional disturbance may adversely attack the spleen; and the reduced warming function of the body due to deficiency of kidney Yang may cause disturbance of metabolism of body fluid to produce diarrhea.

Differential Diagnosis and Treatment

1) Diarrhea caused by damp – heat

The patients may suffer from abdominal pain, prompt diarrhea with yellow and foul stool or with a feeling of incomplete defecation, a burning sensation in anus, a hot feeling and annoyance in the body, thirst and short stream of dark urine. The tongue proper is red in color with yellow and greasy coating and the pulse is soft and rapid or rolling and rapid.

Therapeutic principle   To clear damp – heat and stop diarrhea.

Principal acupoints   **Dàchángdiǎn** and **Fùxièdiǎn**.

Supplemental acupoints   **Sānjiāodiǎn, Xiǎochángdiǎn**.

Xianglian Pills may be orally administered.

2) Diarrhea caused by cold and dampness

The patients may suffer from abdominal pain, diarrhea with thin or watery stool, abdominal distension, distress in upper abdomen, abdominal coldness, poor appetite and long stream of clear urine. The tongue proper is pale with thin, white and greasy coating and the pulse is deep and moderate.

Therapeutic principle   To warm coldness and resolve turbid fluid.

Principal acupoints   **Sānjiāodiǎn** and **Dàchángdiǎn**. The moxibustion with ginger is applied to **Dàchángdiǎn** with moxa cones in a size of a pit of date and changed for 5 times; the hot decoction of fresh ginger 15 g and old tea leaves 10 g may be orally administered in combination to produce a better therapeutic result.

3) Diarrhea due to stagnation of liver qi

The patients may suffer from distension of chest and flank, belching, reduction of food intake, diarrhea and abdominal pain induced by emotional disturbance. The tongue proper is pale with thin and white coating and the pulse is wiry.

Therapeutic principle   To disperse liver qi, adjust spleen and stop diarrhea.

Principal acupoints   **Hégǔ(LI4)** and **Dàchángdiǎn**.

Supplemental   acupoints   **Fùxièdiǎn**,   **Pídiǎn**, **Sānjiāodiǎn**.

4) Diarrhea due to deficiency and weakness of spleen and stomach

The patients may suffer from diarrhea with stool containing undigested food, abdominal distension and sensitiveness to coldness, sallow complexion and weakness of limbs. The tongue proper is pale with thin and white coating and the pulse is thready and weak.

Therapeutic principle   To adjust spleen and stomach and tonify qi.

Principal acupoints   **Pídiǎn** and **Dàchángdiǎn**.

Supplemental   acupoints   **Zúsānlǐ** (ST36), **Xiǎochángdiǎn, Sānjiāodiǎn**. The moxibustion with furnace soil or atractylodes is applied to **Pídiǎn** and **Sānjiāodiǎn** with moxa cones in a size of a pit of date and changed for 3 times until the local skin is flushed. The moxibustion may be also applied to **Shèndiǎn** in patients with early morning diarrhea, abdominal pain and increased intestinal gurgling sound.

5) Diarrhea due to deficiency of kidney Yang

The patients may suffer from cold body and limbs, mental tiredness and early morning diarrhea with stool immediately passed out after the appearance of intestinal gurgling sound and with abdominal pain immediately relieved after the bowel movement. The tongue proper is pale with white coating and the pulse is deep and thready or thready and feeble.

Therapeutic principle   To warm kidney, strengthen spleen, astringe intestine and stop diarrhea.

Principal acupoints　**Nèiguān(PC6)** and **Dàchángdiǎn**.

Supplemental acupoints　**Gōngsūn(SP4)**, **Hégǔ(LI4)**, **Sānjiāodiǎn** and **Shèndiǎn**.

Proctoptosis

Proctoptosis, also commonly known as "prolapse of rectum", is a pathological phenomenon of displacement and prolapse of the rectum and anal canal or even a part of the sigmoid colon, most commonly seen in children, old people, multiparae and weak youngsters and the middle aged.

Etiology and Pathogenesis

The anus is the terminal orifice of colon, which is an exterointeriorly correlated organ of lung. The kidney controls the discharge of urine and stool. If the lung and kidney qi is deficient, the openings of digestive tract may fail to close. The spleen is in charge of digestion and transportation to control the reception of food and discharge of feces. If this function is imperiled due to deficiency and descent of spleen qi, the anus may lose its function to control defecation and the rectum may dropped out of the anus. This disease is common in children with deficiency of qi and blood or in aged people with reduction of qi and blood. It may also occur in patients with deficiency of qi and poor contracting power of anus caused by habitual constipation, chronic diarrhea and dysentery or due to operation of rectum and anus.

Main Points of Diagnosis

1. Most of the patients have a long history of diarrhea.

2. There are two kinds of prolapses. If there is only prolapse of the mucosa and the prolapsed part only protrudes a bit outside with radial plicae, it is called partial prolapse or incomplete prolapse. If the prolapse happens to be of the whole layer of rectum wall or the prolapsed part is rather long with circular folds, it is known as complete prolapse.

3. First, measure the length and the thickness of the prolapsed part. Next, palpate the prolapsed lump to see whether there is a reflected groove or not. After that, determine the size of the "concentric circles" on the top part of the prolapsed lump. Through digital examination with repetition tests make sure of the sphincter strength and so on.

Differential Diagnosis and Treatment

1) Descending of spleen and stomach qi

The rectum may drop out of the anus during walking or after bowel movement and it may or may not be spontaneously reduced. The patients may also have a sensation of tenesmus and a persistent desire to pass stool, a sallow complexion, poor appetite and shortness of breath. The tongue proper is pale with thin white coating and the pulse is wiry.

Therapeutic principle   To elevate and tonify spleen qi.

Principal acupoints   **Zúsānlǐ(ST36)** and **Dàchángdiǎn**.

Supplemental acupoints   **Sānjiāodiǎn, Pídiǎn** and **Xiǎochángdiǎn**.

The moxibustion with ginger and powder of Chinese gall is applied to **Pídiǎn** and **Sānjiāodiǎn** with moxa cones in a size of a pit of Chinese date. Changed for 5 times.

2) Deficiency of spleen and kidney qi

The prolapse of rectum with a small amount of blood and mucus is difficult to replace in severe cases. The patients may also suffer from tenesmus, hatred of coldness, loose stool and long stream of clear urine. The tongue proper is pale with thin and white coating and the pulse is deep and thready or thready and weak.

Therapeutic principle   To strengthen kidney and tonify kidney qi.

Principal acupoints   **Shèndiǎn** and **Dàchángdiǎn**.

Supplemental acupoints   **Sānjiāodiǎn, Guīlái(ST29)**.

Decoction of Chinese gall may be used to wash the anus.

3) Treatment according to the stage of this disease

(1) Early stage

The rectum may drop out of anus after bowel movement and it may be spontaneously replaced. The acupuncture with method of respiratory reduction and reinforcement can be applied at **Dàchángdiǎn, Zhōngwǎn** (RN12) and **Guīlái** (**ST**29).

(2) Middle stage

The manual replacement is necessary to reduce the prolapse of rectum in patients with constant sensation of tenesmus. The acupuncture is applied at **Sānjiāodiǎn, Zhōngwǎn** (**RN**12) and **Tàixī**(**KI**3); and the moxibustion with atractylodes is applied to **Gōngsūn**(**SP**4) with moxa cone changed for 5 times.

(3) Late stage

The rectum may drop out of the anus during standing, walking or coughing and the prolapse of rectum may be stained with some blood and can not be spontaneously replaced. The acupuncture with respiratory reinforcing method or occasionally with reducing method is applied at **Nèiguān** (**PC**6), **Hégǔ**(**LI**4), **Dàchángdiǎn**; the paste of castor bean may be applied over **Yǒngquán**(**KI**1); and the patent herbal drugs, such as Buzhong Yiqi Pills, Shenqi Pills or Suoquan Pills may be administered by mouth according to the nature of disease.

Constipation

Constipation refers to difficulty in defecation and prolonged interval between every two courses of defecation. It is
responsible for prolonged retention of feces in the intestine.
This long retention gets feces over – dried and hard to be discharged.

Etiology and Pathogenesis

The excessive constipation usually occurs in patients
with excessive Yang in the body and accumulation of heat
pathogen in stomach and intestine after intake of much spicy
and fried food and at the same time attacked by external heat
pathogen; but the deficient constipation usually occurs in
aged people with deficiency of liver and kidney essence and
accumulation of cold pathogen in intestine or in patients with
chronic diseases or in women after childbirth due to loss of

moisturizing and lubricating materials in intestine.

Differential Diagnosis and Treatment

1) Excessive constipation

The patients may suffer from constipation, abdominal distension, preference of coolness and hatred of hotness, dark urine and dryness in mouth with desire to drink water. The tongue proper is red in color with yellow and dry coating and the pulse is full and rapid.

Therapeutic principle   To promote flow of qi in hollow organs and clear dry heat.

Principal acupoints   **Dàchángdiǎn** and **Hégǔ(LI4)**.

Supplemental acupoints   **Pídiǎn, Zhīgōu (SJ6)** and **Shèndiǎn**.

2) Deficient constipation

. The patients may suffer from constipation, physical and mental tiredness, sallow complexion, dizziness, palpitation of heart, cold limbs, no strength to pass stool and frequent urination. The tongue proper is pale with white coating and the pulse is deep and thready.

Therapeutic principle   To tonify Yin, moisten dryness, tonify qi and strengthen spleen.

Principal acupoints   **Dàchángdiǎn, Guānyuán (RN4)** and **Zhīgōu(SJ6)**.

Supplemental   acupoints   **Shàoshāng (LU11)**,

Xiǎochángdiǎn, Zhāngmén(LR13) and Yángchí(SJ4).

The acupuncture with reducing technique is used to treat excessive constipation; and the acupuncture with reinforcing technique along with moxibustion is used to treat deficient constipation. In addition to acupuncture, the massage over abdomen may help the bowel movement.

Migraine

The migraine is a disease with pain on one side of head, usually occurred after tiredness.

Etiology and Pathogenesis

The pathogenic organs of migraine are liver and gall-bladder and the pathogenic factors are stagnation of phlegm, fire and blood or invasion of external wind pathogen. One function of the liver is in charge of dispersing liver qi. If the gallbladder meridian is obstructed and the meridional qi can not freely flow or the liver blood is deficient to nourish the meridian, migraine occurs.

Differential Diagnosis and Treatment

The patient may suffer from severe pain on one side of the head, poor appetite, tastelessness in mouth and distention in the chest and upper abdomen. The onset of headache is often induced by emotional disturbance and the women may have severe migraine with pulsation of blood vessels during menstrual period or at the late stage. The tongue proper is pale with thin and white coating and the pulse is wiry and thready or thready and weak.

Therapeutic principle   To disperse liver qi, promote the discharge of bile and remove stasis in collaterals.

Principal acupoints   **Piāntóudiǎn, Hòutóudiǎn** and **Hégǔ(LI4)**.

Supplemental acupoints   **Gāndiǎn, Shàochōng(HT9)**.

Yānhóudiǎn and **Sānjiāodiǎn** may be added to treat patients with bitter taste in mouth, dryness in throat and vertigo due to accumulation of heat in liver and gallbladder; **Xiōngdiǎn** and **Sānjiāodiǎn** may be added to treat patients with fullness and distention in the chest and upper abdomen due to accumulation of phlegm and dampness; **Shèndiǎn** may be added to treat migraine during menstruation; **Yǎndiǎn** may be added to treat headache with eye incapable of opening; and **Qiántóudiǎn** may be added to treat pain in the frontal area of the head.

Insomnia

The symptom insomnia refers to prolonged and usually abnormal inability to obtain adequate sleep. Some patients may complain of the difficulty in falling asleep; some are easy to be awakened, but can not fall asleep again; some patients may have an intermittent sleep discontinued from time to time; and the patients with severe insomnia may be sleepless throughout a whole night and even day by day through months.

Etiology and Pathogenesis

The pathogenic factors of insomnia are either deficiency of vital energy or excessiveness of pathogens. The heart is an organ to control blood circulation and mental activity and the spleen can produce blood and adjust thinking process. The worriment may consume blood and cause deficiency of heart and spleen and pregnancy and childbirth of women may also cause deficiency of blood and injure heart and spleen. There-fore, they are the main pathogenic factors of insomnia, on account of which the heart can not obtain enough nourish-ment. The congenital deficiency of essence and loss of essence in patients indulgent in sexual activity are also the pathogenic factors of insomnia. In chronic patients with wasting of Yin, the poor communication between heart and kidney due to deficiency of Yin and excessiveness of fire pathogen may also cause insomnia. In excessive type of in-somnia, the disturbance of sleep may be caused by accumula-tion of phlegm and fire pathogen or dysfunction of stomach.

Differential Diagnosis and Treatment

1) Deficient type of insomnia

(1) Deficiency of heart and spleen   The patients may have a dreamy sleep easily awakened, poor memory, palpita-tion of heart, sallow complexion, mental tiredness and taste-lessness in mouth. The tongue proper is pale with white coating and the pulse is thready and weak.

Therapeutic principle   To enrich nutrients, tonify blood and tranquilize mind.

Principal acupoints   **Xīndiǎn, Shèndiǎn,** and **Pídiǎn**.

Supplemental acupoints   **Láogōng (PC8), Nèiguān (PC6)**.

(2) Deficiency of Yin and excessiveness of fire pathogen

The patients may suffer from insomnia, annoyance, vertigo, tinnitus, dryness in mouth with scanty saliva, or emission of semen and lumbago. The tongue proper is red in color with scanty coating and the pulse is thready and rapid.

Therapeutic principle   To tonify water (Yin) and reduce fire (Yang) and to promote communication of heart and kidney.

Principal acupoints   **Láogōng (PC8), Shàofǔ (HT8), Shèndiǎn** and **Xīndiǎn**.

Supplemental acupoints   **Gāndiǎn**. **Gāndiǎn** added for deficiency of gallbladder qi.

2) Excessive type of insomnia

(1) Dysfunction of stomach   The patients may suffer from unsteady sleep, distension of upper abdomen, belching, dizziness and vertigo. The tongue proper is red in color with thin and white coating and the pulse is rolling.

Therapeutic principle   To improve digestion, regulate stomach and tranquilize mind.

Principal acupoints   **Pídiǎn** and **Láogōng(PC8)**.

Supplemental   acupoints   **Shàofǔ (HT8)**   and **Xiǎochángdiǎn**.

(2) Accumulation of phlegm and fire pathogen   The patients may suffer from vertigo, bitter taste in mouth, chest distress with much sputum, annoyance and bad temper. The

coating is yellow and greasy and the pulse is rolling and rapid. They may suffer from sleeplessness throughout a whole night, red eyes, dryness in mouth, annoyance and hotness in the chest, constipation and short stream of dark urine. The tongue proper is red in color with yellow coating and the pulse is wiry and rolling.

Therapeutic principle   To resolve phlegm and clear heat.

Principal acupoints   **Wèichángtòngdiǎn, Shèndiǎn** and **Pídiǎn**.

Supplemental acupoints   **Shàofǔ(HT8), Yújì(LU10), Láogōng(PC8)** and **Fèidiǎn**.

Sleepiness

The patients with sleepiness may be always sleepy and drowsy day and night. After awakened by other person, they may quickly fall asleep again and in severe cases, the sleepiness is very difficult to improve.

Etiology and Pathogenesis

The important pathogenic factors of this disease are deficiency of Yang, excessiveness of Yin, deficiency of spleen, excessiveness of dampness pathogen and blockage of circulation of Yang. The property of Yang is active and dynamic; and the property of Yin is stable and static. The patients may be spiritless due to deficiency of Yang and can not open eyes due to excessiveness of Yin. As mentioned in Miraculous Pivot: "The eyes may open wide if Yang is excessive; and the eyes are closed, if Yin is excessive."

Differential Diagnosis and Treatment

Symptoms   Weakness of limbs, sleepiness after meal, chest distress, reduced intake of food and long – lasting sleepiness.

Signs   The tongue proper is pale with thin and white coating and the pulse is deep.

Therapeutic principle   To support Yang and suppress Yin.

Principal acupoint   **Láogōng(PC**8).

Supplemental acupoints   **Shèndiǎn, Gāndiǎn, Sānjiāodiǎn** and **Yángchí(SJ**4). The moxibustion with grass – leaved sweetflag rhizome is applied at **Yángchí(SJ**4) with moxa cones in a size of a pit of date and is changed for 5 times.

Palpitation

The symptom palpitation, or frightening and palpitation of heart in traditional Chinese medicine, is a subjective symptom with unstable mood and increased heart beats. The frightening is an exogenous symptom and palpitation of the heart is an endogenous one and the latter is more serious than the former. However, they have a similar etiology and pathogenesis.

Etiology and Pathogenesis

The frightening and palpitation of the heart is related to some mental factors and is caused by deficiency of heart blood and unsteadiness of mind. The pathogenic organ of this symptom is the heart which can control the mental activity. The heart can also control blood and blood vessels. The heart may lose the supply of nutrients from blood and the mental activity may be disturbed if the blood is deficient. The heart fire may be exacerbated to disturb the mental activity if the kidney water (Yin) is insufficient to nourish the heart. The upward attack of turbid fluid pathogen may block and inhibit heart Yang to produce palpitation of heart. The deficiency of qi of heart and gallbladder may cause frightening. The heart blood may also be wasted by extreme tiredness of mind to cause this symptom.

Differential Diagnosis and Treatment

1) Deficiency of heart blood

The patients may suffer from dizziness, vertigo, pale complexion, palpitation of heart and unsteady sleep with frightening. The tongue proper is pink in color with thin coating and the pulse is thready and weak.

Therapeutic principle   To tonify blood and tranquilize mind.

Principal acupoints   **Xīndiǎn, Láogōng (PC8), Xiōngdiǎn**.

Supplemental acupoints   **Pídiǎn, Nèiguān (PC6), Hégǔ(LI4), Yángchí(SJ4)**.

2) Deficiency of Yin and excessiveness of fire pathogen

The patients suffer from frightening and palpitation of heart, hotness evil in the heart, feverish sensation in the palms and soles, vertigo, tinnitus and dryness in mouth without desire to drink water. The tongue proper is red in color with scanty coating and the pulse is thready and rapid.

Therapeutic principle   To tonify Yin and clear fire.

Principal acupoints   **Xīndiǎn, Nèiguān (PC6)** and **Shénmén(HT7)**.

Supplemental acupoints   **Shèndiǎn, Yújì (LU10), Shàofǔ(HT8)** and **Láogōng(PC8)**.

3) Deficiency of qi of heart and gallbladder

The patients may suffer from frightening and palpitation of the heart, annoyance, unsteadiness of mind in any posture, dreaminess and easy awakening, tastelessness in the mouth, and poor appetite. The tongue proper is red in color with thin and yellow coating and the pulse is wiry and moderate.

Therapeutic principle   To warm gallbladder and tonify qi of thegallbladder, release frightening and tranquilize mind.

Principal acupoints   **Nèiguān (PC6), Gāndiǎn** and **Xīndiǎn**.

Supplemental acupoints   **Yángchí (SJ4), Wàiguān (SJ5), Láogōng(PC8), Shàofǔ(HT8)**.

Xiong Bi

Xiong bi, or Bi − syndrome of chest is a disease with chest distress and pain, which may be radiated to the back. The severe patients may suffer from colic pain in chest with shortness of breath.

Etiology and Pathogenesis

In patient with deficiency of Yang, the external cold pathogen may attack the chest to cause blockage of circulation of Yang in chest. The endogenous phlegm and dampness may block the spread of Yang qi in the chest and even cause stagnation of qi and blood in chronic cases.

Differential Diagnosis and Treatment

The patients with mild manifestations only have chest distress and unsmooth breath; and the severe patients may suffer from chest pain radiated to back, asthma and shortness of breath. The onset of chest pain may be very prompt together with pale complexion, cold limbs and sweating. The pulse is feeble.

1) Deficient and cold type

The patients may have chillness and cold limbs and the disease can be deteriorated by the attack of cold pathogen.

Therapeutic principle   To promote circulation of Yang qi, expel cold pathogen, warm and tonify qi and promote circulation of qi.

Principal acupoints   **Xīndiǎn** and **Nèiguān(PC6)** and **Mìngméndiǎn**.

Supplemental acupoint   **Yángchí(SJ4)**.

2) Phlegm and turbid fluid type

The patients may have cough with profuse sputum.

Therapeutic principle   To strengthen spleen, resolve phlegm, remove chest distrees and adjust circulation of qi.

Principal acupoints   **Pídiǎn** and **Fèidiǎn**.

Supplemental acupoint   **Xiǎochángdiǎn**.

3) Blood stagnation type

The patients may have pricking chest pain, purple lips and dark tongue.

Therapeutic principle   To promote circulation of qi, blood and Yang in order to stop pain.

Principal acupoints **Xīndiǎn** and **Yángchí**(SJ4).

Supplemental acupoints **Shèndiǎn** and **Sānjiāodiǎn**.

The balanced reinforce − reducing technique is used for application of acupuncture at all acupoints; and the moxibustion and cupping therapy may be used to treat patients of first two types.

Hysteria

Hysteria is a psychoneurosis marked by emotional excitability and disturbance of the psychic, sensory, vasomotor, and visceral functions without an organic basis. It is a common neurotic disease in youths with functional disturbance of brain caused by some mental factors. This disease has a prompt onset, high suggestibility, quick curability and short clinical course.

Etiology and Pathogenesis

The heart is in charge of mental activity; the liver can store blood and has a function to disperse qi; the kidney can store essence and deal with ideal; and the kidney essence can produce bone marrow and the brain is a reservoir of bone marrow to deal with spirit. The essence of all internal organs and Yang qi in all meridians may assemble into the brain. The brain may lose its nutrition and fail to adjust mental activity, if the heart blood and kidney essence are deficient and the Ying (nutritive materials) and Wei (defensive energy) are disturbed. The liver may lose its dispersing function and the brain may lose its function to adjust mental activity after they are damaged by emotional disturbance to produce high mental irritability and restless physical movement.

Differential Diagnosis and Treatment

1) Exuberant liver and weakened spleen

The patients may have unstable mood, high irritability and angry, violent rage, distension and pain of flank and costal region from time to time, vomiting, belching, obstructing sensation in throat, distension and pain in upper abdomen, convulsion and no desire to take food, speak and move. The tongue coating is white in color and the pulse is wiry and thready.

Therapeutic principle　To adjust function of liver and spleen and tranquilize mind.

Principal acupoints　**Láogōng (PC8)** and **Yángchí (SJ4)**.

Supplemental acupoints　**Gāndiǎn, Sānjiāodiǎn, Hégǔ (LI4)** and **Zhōngchōng(PC9)**.

2) Deficiency of liver and kidney Yin

The patients may suffer from dizziness, insomnia and

dreaminess, emission of semen, hotness in heart, palms and soles, tinnitus, obstruction of ear, blindness, palpitation of heart, mental confusion, tremor, dryness in mouth, unreasonable dance for joy and uncortrollable laugh. The tongue proper is red in color with scanty coating and the pulse is wiry and thready or thready and rapid.

Therapeutic principle   To enrich Yin and tranquilize mind.

Principal acupoint   **Láogōng (PC8)**, **Xīndiǎn** and **Gāndiǎn**.

3) Accumulation of phlegm and heat pathogen

The patients may suffer from aphasia, mental depression, paraplegia, hemiplegia, intentional closure of eyes and mouth, flushed face, rough breath, artificial rigidity of whole body and purposely holding breath. The pulse is wiry and rapid or rolling and rapid.

Therapeutic principle   To resolve phlegm, release stasis of collaterals and open orifices of sense organs.

Principal acupoint   **Láogōng(PC8)**

Supplemental acupoints   **Shàofǔ (HT8)**, **Zhōngchōng (PC9)** and **Wèichángtòngdiǎn**. The reducing technique is applied to all acupoints.

Body acupuncture

Prescription   **Shuǐgōu(DU26)**, **Hégǔ(LI4)**, **Tàichōng (LR3)**.

Supplementary points   For liver - qi stagnation, **Yánglíngquán(GB34)** and **Dǎnzhōng(RN17)** are added; for insufficiency of blood, **Jiūwěii(RN15)** and **Nèiguān(PC6)**.

Method   Use filiform needles to puncture the points with reducing method.

Auricular acupuncture

Prescription   Gan (CO_{12}) liver, Xin (CO_{15}) heart, Shenmen(TF_4) shenmen, Pizhixia(AT_4) subcortex, Jiaogan (AH_{6a}) sympathetic nerve, Zhen(AT_3) occiput.

Method   Use filiform needles to puncture the points with strong twirling and rotating method for continuous five minutes and retain them for 30 to 40 minutes. The needles are not withdrawn until the symptoms disappear and the patient feels easy.

Epilepsy

Epilepsy is defined as paroxysmal and temporary disturbance of brain characterized by loss of consciousness and muscle tic abnormal sensation, emotion and behavior. In traditional Chinese medicine, this disease is categorized as "Xian Zheng" (epilepsy syndrome) and "Dian Xian" (epilepsy).

Etiology and Pathogenesis

Epilepsy may have many causes. It is often associated with phlegm. As the saying goes: "No epilepsy develops without phlegm."

1. Congenital factors   Disturbance of qi and blood of a mother caused by great terror may affect her fetus who may develop epilepsy after birth. Besides, congenital insufficiency of liver – yin and kidney – yin, imbalance of water and fire, impairment of heart and liver are all responsible for disturbance of liver – qi, for mental derangement, convulsion and

loss of consciousness. The acquired epilepsy of infants due to frightening is also associated with congenital factors. All that are induced by terror are called convulsive diseases.

2. Blockage of Phlegm in Orifices　There is usually excessive phlegm in infants due to retention of dampness caused by hypofunction of the spleen. Besides, retention of wind and phlegm may still stay in the body after chronic or acute infantile convulsion. It is the accumulation of phlegm in the interior when precipitated by wind, cold or terror, that attacks the upper orifices, therefore inducing epilepsy.

3. Retention of Food in the Middle – Jiao　Improper feeding, or excessive greasy and sweet foods may all be responsible for the impariment of the spleen and stomach. The dsiorder of receiptive and digestive functions, thus developing infantile dyspepsia. A prolonged retention may transform pathogenic heat, consuming body fluid to from phlegm. Stagnation of phlegm in the middle – jiao makes spleen – qi fails to ascend and stomach – qi to descend.

4. Blood Stasis in the Heart　Accumulation of blood stasis in the heart may be caused by events of birth injury, terror, trauma, or head injury, which may lead mental confusion into epilepsy.

Main Points of Diagnosis

1. The histories of family, epileptic attack and en-

cephalopathia should be inquired carefully.

2. Clinical manifestations of the disease vary greatly. There may be grand mal, petit mal, rolandic mal and infantile spasms. The grand mal is cahracterized by sudden loss of consciousness, general totanic spasm with apnea, cyanosis and foam in the mouth, which usually last for 1 − 5 minutes. The patients may then fall into sleep and become conscious a few hours later. The petit mal is characterized by sudden, short loss of consciousness without aurae and muscle tic, accompanied with interruptions of speech and action which usually persisrt for 2 − 10 seconds. The patient usually comes to consciousness rapidly.

3. Electroencephalogram examination and tomography may be useful for the diagnosis of epilepsy. During the episode of epilepsy, the patients may suddenly fall down with loss of consciousness, upward staring of eyes, convulsion of limbs, overflowing of foamy saliva and strange screaming. Then they may completely recover after a short period of attack and quickly restore their normal daily life without any sequelae.

Differential Diagnosis and Treatment

1) During the attack of epilepsy

At the beginning, the patients may have dizziness, vertigo, headache and chest distress; then they may fall down and develop mental confusion, upward staring of eyes, convulsion of limbs and overflowing of foamy saliva; and finally they may restore their normal mentality and daily life. The tongue coating is white and greasy and the pulse is wiry and rolling; or the tongue coating is yellow and greasy and the pulse is rolling and rapid.

Therapeutic principle To resolve phlegm, control wind and open orifices of sense organs.

Principal acupoints **Láogōng (PC8), Hégǔ (LI4), Nèiguān(PC6).**

Supplemental acupoints **Yángchí (SJ4), Shàochōng (HT9), Zhōngchōng(PC9), Shèndiǎn, Gāndiǎn.** The reducing technique is applied with the needles not retained.

2) After attack of epilepsy

After the attack of epilepsy, the vital energy of the patients must be deficient, so that the vital energy should be enriched to prevent the relapse.

(1) Deficiency of spleen and kidney

The patients may suffer from mental tiredness, sallow complexion, dizziness, lumbago, profuse sputum and poor appetite. The tongue proper is pale with white coating and the pulse is thready and rolling.

Therapeutic principle To tonify kidney and spleen.

Principal acupoints **Pídiǎn** and **Yángchí(SJ4).**

Supplemental acupoints **Sānjiāodiǎn, Shèndiǎn.**

Pídiǎn and **Sānjiāodiǎn** are heated with moxa cones made from atractylodes in a size of a pit of date and changed for 5 times.

(2) Deficiency of essence and blood

The patients may suffer from spiritlessness, sallow complexion, dizziness, palpitation of heart, soreness of waist, soreness and weakness of leg. The tongue proper is pale and the pulse is feeble and weak.

Therapeutic principle　　To tonify blood and essence.

Principal acupoints　　**Nèiguān** (PC6) and **Láogōng** (PC8).

Supplemental acupoints　　**Yángchí** (SJ4), **Gāndiǎn**, **Shèndiǎn** and **Xīndiǎn**.

The dry powder of placenta 10 g may be orally administered 3 times a day for a long time; and the Dianxian Powde 10 g 3 times a day may be administered to the patients with profuse sputum.

Peripheral Facial Paralysis
(Bell's Palsy)

Bell's palsy is a paralysis of one side of the face, is facial paralysis which occurs suddenly and mostly after exposure to cold wind or trauma. It may occur at any age but is slightly more common in the age group from 20 to 50. 85 – 90% of the patients get recovered spontaneously. In traditional Chinese medicine, the onset of the illness is thought to be due to derangement of qi and blood and malnutrition of the channels caused by invasion of the channels and collaterals in the facial region by pathogenic wind – cold or phlegm. If falls into the category of "zhen zhong feng", "kou yan wai xie" or "diao xian feng" (deviation of the eye and mouth) in traditional Chinese medicine.

Etiology and Pathogenesis

The paralysis of facial muscles is caused by the attack of

wind cold or wind heat pathogen to the meridians of face and the stagnation of qi in meridians or due to the invasion of damp – heat pathogen from liver and gallbladder to the meridians.

Main Points of Diagnosis

1. It often occurs in autumn and winter or between spring and summer, mostly in the middle – aged. The disease usually attacks one side of the face.

2. The diagnosis is based on the symptoms, but most rule out cerebrovascular accidents (strokes) and intracranial tumors. The peripheral facial paralysis patients are specially unable to frown and raise the eyebrow, close the eye of the paralyzed side. The intracranial tumors can be ruled out X – ray examination.

3. The attack comes all of a sudden. At the beginning the patient feels numb at one side of the face, pain around the ear and tenderness in the mastoidal region. Then the mouth becomes wry, the nasolabial groove no longer seen and the facio – buccal region relaxed and strengthless. It is impossible to have the cheeks blown up. The eyeballs are still exposed when the eyes are shut. It is difficult to frown and speak. Salivation comes down from the corners of the mouth. The sense of taste is lost but the sense of hearing is hypersensitive. There may be pain in the mastoid region or

headache.

Differential Diagnosis and Treatment

1) Wind heat pathogen

The patients may suffer from headache, deviation of mouth and eye, lacrimation, dripping of saliva, fever, chillness, burning pain and redness in ear root, annoyance, dryness and bitter taste in mouth, dark urine and constipation. The tongue proper is red in color with yellow and greasy coating and the pulse is floating and rapid.

Therapeutic principle   To expel wind, clear heat and release stasis in collaterals.

Principal acupoints   **Hégǔ(LI4)** and **Qiántóudiǎn**.

Supplemental acupoints   **Shāngyáng (LI1)**, **Láogōng (PC8)**.

2) Wind cold pathogen

The patients may suffer from deviation of mouth and eye, hatred of coldness to face, pale complexion, severe pain in the ear root, headache, poor appetite and long stream of clear urine. The tongue proper is pale with thin and white coating and the pulse is floating and tense.

Therapeutic principle   To expel wind and cold pathogen and release stasis in the collaterals.

Principal acupoints   **Yángchí(SJ4)**, **Shàofǔ(HT8)**.

Supplemental acupoints   **Nèiguān** (PC6), **Wàiguān** (SJ5).

Body Acupuncture Therapy

Points   **Yìfēng**(SJ17), **Dìcāng**(ST4), **Jiáchē**(ST6), **Yángbái**(GB14), **Tàiyáng** (EX − HN5), **Hégǔ** (LI4), **Quánliáo**(SI18) and **Xiàguān**(ST7).

Method   3 to 5 of the above points are selected for each treatment and the therapy is given once daily. **Dìcāng**(ST4) and **Jiáchē**(ST6) are punctured together with one needle inserted horizontally from **Dìcāng**(ST4) to **Jiáchē**(ST6). The following points can also be added to the formula according to the symptoms: **Fēngchí** (GB20) for headache; **Fēnglóng** (ST40) for profuse sputum; **Cuánzhú**(BL2) and **Sīzhúkōng** (SJ23) for difficulty in frowning and raising the eyebrow; **Cuánzhú**(BL2), **Jīngmíng**(BL1), **Tóngzǐliáo**(GB1), **Yúyāo** (EX − HN4) and **Sīzhúkōng**(SJ23) for incomplete closing of the eyelids; **Yíngxiāng** (LI20) for difficulty in sniffing; **Shuǐgōu**(DU26) for deviation of the philtrum; **Jūliáo**(GB29) for inability to show the teeth; **Tīnghuì**(GB2) for tinnitus and deafness; **Wàngǔ**(SI4) for tenderness at the mastoid region; and **Tàichōng**(LR3) for twitching of the eyelid and the mouth.

Electro − acupuncture Therapy

Main Points   **Qianzheng**(an extra − point) and **Yìfēng** (SJ17).

Auxiliary Points　**Yángbái**(**GB**14), **Tàiyáng**(**EX** − **HN**5) **and Dìcāng**(**ST**4).

Method　One of the main points and two or three of the auxiliary points are prescribed each time. The main point is connected to the negative pole of the electro − acupuncture machine, and the auxiliary points to the positive pole. The frequency is adjusted to 20 to 30 times per minute with an output which can just cause the muscular twitch on the affected side. The treatment lasts for 15 minutes and is repeated once every other day. Ten times consisted of one course.

The patient can be assured that recovery usually occurs in 2 to 8 weeks (or up to one to two years in older patients). In the vast majority of cases, partial or complete recovery occurs. When recovery is partial, contractures may develop on the paralyzed side. Recurrence on the same or the opposite side is occasionally reported.

Other External Treatment

1) Apply adhesive plaster on the acupoints　Dust 0.5 to 1 gram of the powder of Semen Strychni onto a plaster and then apply the plaster on the acupoint of **Tàiyáng**(**EX** − **HN**5), **Xiàguān**(**ST**7) and **Jiáchē**(**ST**6) of the affected side (more applicable to the regions with tenderness). Change the plaster every 3 days. If blisters appear on the administered part, extract its fluid after disinfection. Then the blisters will get cured spontaneously.

2) Smear the blood of eel onto the affected region

Smear fresh blood of eel onto the buccal skin of the affected side, and hold the mouth angle of the affected side with a metal hook so as to help cure the facial paralysis. This is to be done once a day.

3) Do local massage on the affected region, several times a day.

Therapeutic Methods by Practising Qigong

1. Self – Treatment by Practising Qigong

1) Basic Maneuvers

It is advisable to practise Head and Face Qigong.

2) Auxiliary Maneuvers

Those shedding tears ought to lay emphasis on kneading **Yángbái(GB14)**, **Sìbái(ST2)**, and **Tóngzǐliáo(GB1)**.

At the initial stage, the pressing and kneading manipulations applied locally should be light; as for those with a long course of disease, the manipulations should be heavier.

2. External Qi Therapy

1) Basic Maneuvers

(1) Press and knead the acupoints **Yángbái (GB14)**, **Chéngqì (ST1)**, **Sīzhúkōng (SJ23)**, **Tóngzǐliáo (GB1)**, **Tīnggōng (SI19)**, **Yìfēng (SJ17)**, **Quánliáo (SI18)**, **Yíngxiāng(LI20) Jiáchē(ST6)**, **Fēngchí(GB20)** and **Hégǔ (LI4)**.

(2) Apply the flat – palm form, use the pushing,

268

Internal Diseases

pulling and leading manipulations to emit qi onto the unilateral paralyzed face, conduct the channel qi from front to back and along the Large Intestine Meridian to the terminals of the upper extremities.

2) Auxiliary Maneuvers

In the anaphase of the paralysis, the additional application of the vibrating and quivering manipulation is advised to provoke the channel qi.

Treatment by Chinese Massage

There will be gradual recovery in on or two weeks after its onset. Manipulation of massage may help the recovery of facial nerves and muscular function and reduce sequelae. During the treatment, stimulus of cold to the face and head should be avoided and the patient should knead the face frequently for enhancing the effectiveness.

1. Manipulation　Pushing with one − finger meditation, digital − pressing, pressing, grasping and kneading.

2. Location of Points: **Hégǔ (LI4)**, **Qūchí (LI11)**, **Xiàguān(ST7)**, **Jiáchē(ST6)**, **Yìfēng(SJ17)**, **Tàiyáng(EX − HN5)**, **Jīngmíng(BL1)**, **Sìbái(ST2)**, **Yíngxiāng(LI20)**, **Shuǐgōu(DU26)** and **Dìcāng(ST4)**.

3. Operation

1) The doctor stands in front and to the side of the sitting patient and holds the posterolateral part of the head with

· 134 ·

one hand. Using one − finger meditation pushing or thumb − pressing − kneading, the doctor pushes with the other hand repeatedly from **Yìntáng**(**EX − HN3**) along the supercilliary of the affected side to **Tàiyáng**(**EX − HN5**) for 2 or 3 times first; then pushes repeatedly from **Yìntáng**(**EX − HN3**) upwards by way of **Shéntíng**(**DU24**) to **Bǎihuì**(**DU20**) also for 2 or 3 times; finally, pushes repeatedly from the middle of the forehead via **Yángbái** (**GB**14) of the affected part to **Tàiyáng**(**EX − HN5**) for 2 or 3 times.

2) After that, in the above − mentioned way, the doctor pushes downwards repeatedly from Yintang(EX − HN3) by way of **Jīngmíng**(**BL1**) of the affected side, along the side of the nose up to **Yingxiang**(**LI20**) for 2 or 3 times. Then the doctor pushes from **Yíngxiāng**(**LI20**), along the point of **Sìbái**(**ST2**), **Quánliáo**(**SI**18), **Xiàguān**(**ST7**) and **Jiáchē** (**ST6**) passing the face, to **Dìcāng**(**ST4**) at the labial angle.

3) Still in the same way mentioned above, the operator pushes from **Dìcāng**(**ST4**) to **Shuǐgōu**(**DU26**) circling the lips, by way of **Chéngjiāng** (**RN24**), and returns to the starting point. Then the operator pushes along the mandible to **Jiáchē**(**ST6**). Finally rub and scrub softly the affected side of the face with the palm till local warmth and heat are produced.

In the above − mentioned operations, the movement of the hand should pass at every point with a bit more strength exerted and some stimulating manipulations such as digit −

pressing used in combination.

4) The doctor stands to the side of the patient and, with one hand holding his forehead, grasps **Fēngchí(GB20)** and the tendons of the back nape up and down repeatedly for three to five times, finally pushes the point Qiaogong for 30 times.

5) The doctor standing behind the patient, grasps **Jiānjǐng(GB21)** with two hands and in an orderly way presses and kneads **Qūchí(LI11)** and **Hégǔ(LI4)**.

4. Course of Treatment   Once a day, six days for one course with an interval of 3 days between two courses.

Trigeminal Neuralgia

Trigeminal neuralgia refers to short paroxysmal attacks of severe spastic pain over the distributing area of trigeminal nerve on the face, usually induced by the hot, cold, sour or spicy stimulation. It is called facial pain in traditional Chinese medicine.

Etiology and Pathogenesis

The foot Yangming, Shaoyang and Taiyang meridians and their meridional muscles pass through the region of face with pain of trigeminal neuralgia, which is caused by the invasion of wind, cold and heat pathogens into those meridians to block the circulation of qi through them. The neuralgic pain may also be caused by the stagnation of liver qi and the change of liver qi to fire after the liver is injured by emotional disturbance, because the liver fire may flame up to scorch the face and to produce pain. In addition, the extraction of tooth, trauma, accumulation of heat pathogen in stomach and stagnation of cold and dampness may also produce this disease. The neuralgic pain may suddenly appear in excessive type; and the chronic and lingering pain on face may appear in deficient type of trigeminal neuralgia. The repeated attacks over years may cause stagnation of qi and blood and deficiency of qi.

Main Points of Diagnosis

1. It is characterized by paroxysmal burning sensation on the face with severe flash pain accompanied with facial spasm and lacrimation which usually last for few seconds and then relieves spontaneously. The patient feels nothing abnormal during interval of attacks.

2. the pain is usually induced by muscular movement of the face and referred to the lips, ala nasi and jaw.

3. Generally, there is no positive symptoms of nerve system.

4. Clinically, it should be differentiated from toothache, sinusitis and glossopharyngeal neuralgia.

Differential Diagnosis and Treatment

Clinical manifestations

The pain of trigeminal neuralgia is limited in the innervating area of trigeminal nerve, more common in the distributing region of second and third branches of this nerve, but it may be spread to other branch following the progress of the disease. During the episode, the severe lightning, cutting and burning pain may suddenly appear and last for several seconds. The times of attack are irregular and varied from few times a day to many times in an hour. The facial pain may cause twitches of facial muscles, flushing of face and lacrimation and redness of eyes. The attacks may be induced by speaking, swallowing, tooth – brushing, face – washing and blowing air. The tenderness may be detected over the supraorbital notch, infraorbital foramen and mental foramen.

Therapeutic principle   To disperse wind, release stasis in collaterals, promote blood circulation and relax muscles.

Principal acupoints   **Hégǔ(LI4)** and **Qiántóudiǎn**.

Supplemental acupoints   **Bāxié (EX – UE9)**, **Sānjiāodiǎn**, **Xiàguān(ST7)**.

The reducing technique is applied at **Bāxié(EX – UE9)**, **Xiàguān(ST7)**; the balanced reinforce – reducing technique is applied at **Sānjiāodiǎn**; the blue dragon swaying tail technique is applied at **Hégǔ(LI4)**; and the acupuncture is applied twice a day and the needles are retained for 30 min.

In patients with trigeminal neuralgia caused by wind and cold pathogens with phlegm, exacerbated by coldness and improved or relieved by hotness, the warm acupuncture may be applied at **Pídiǎn** and **Sānjiāodiǎn** for 30 min.

In patients of trigeminal neuralgia with local sweating caused by wind and heat pathogens, exacerbated by hotness and improved or relieved by coldness, **Shàozé(SI1)** may be used; and the bleeding therapy may be applied at **Bāxié(EX −UE9)**.

In patients of trigeminal neuralgia with flushing face caused by liver fire, **Láogōng(PC8)** and **Shàofǔ(HT8)** may be used to reduce liver fire.

Sciatica

Sciatica refers to the pain in the passage ways of the sciatic nerve and its distribution region, radiating from the buttock along the posterior part of the thigh and the posterolateral portion of the shank to the distal portion. It is mainly caused by sciatic neuritis and the changes of the adjacent structures, belonging to the categories of "Bi Zheng" (arthralgia – syndrome) and "Yao Tui Tong" (pain in the waist and lower extemities) in traditional Chinese medicine.

Etiology and Pathogenesis

The neuralgia sciatica caused by coldness and infection can be divided into primary and secondary types. The primary neuralgia sciatica is a disease of the sciatic nerve itself; but the secondary neuralgia sciatica is caused by the lesions in nearby structures and tissues of sciatic nerve, including prolapse of intervertebral disc, lumbar hypertrophic spondylitis, arthritis of spinal column, intraspinal tumor and diseases of iliosacral joint and pelvis. In traditional Chinese medicine, the neuralgia sciatica belongs to Bi − syndrome. If caused by wind pathogen, the pain may wander here and there or may be radiated up and down; if caused by dampness pathogen, the pain may linger for a long time and fix at a defined area; and if caused by cold pathogen, the pain is very severe. In addition, the deficiency of liver and kidney Yin and poor nutrition of meridians may also produce this disease.

Main Symptoms and Signs

At the beginning of the disease, there is usually a lateral pain in the waist and with the development of the disease the pain radiates suddenly or gradually along the buttock of the affected side, the posterior aspect of the thigh and the posterolateral side of the leg and the dorsum of the foot or the lateral margin of foot. And a burning, lancinating or electric − shock like pain may appear along the spreading area of the sciatic nerve. At the beginning, the pain is mostly paroxysmal, increases after tiredness, disappears after rest, and becomes severe and continuous gradually afterwards. Usually there is septal repeated attack which may last several weeks, several months or even several years. On examination, the physiological curvature of the lumbar vertebrae can be seen as flat and straight, or the lateral curvature and the lumbar muscle may look tense. And near the spinous process of the affected side of the lumbar vertebrae there is a distinct tenderness point which radiates towards the lower limbs of the affected side. The test of straight leg – raising is positive. Neck flexion and neck pressure test are also positive. In a long – standing case, there may be hypoesthesia or anesthesia or muscular atrophy of the affected limb.

Types of Syndromes

1. Arthralgia – syndrome due to Wind – Cold – Dampness

Pain in the waist and lower extremities, inability to bend, stretch, toss or turn which is aggravated in overcast and rainy weather, heaviness, numbness and cold sensation of the affected region, whitish greasy coating of the tongue, taut pulse.

2. Deficiency of the Liver and Kidney

Pain in the waist and lower extremities, soreness and weakness of the waist and knees, pain and numbness of the affected region, listlessness, thin whitish coating of the tongue, deep thready and feeble pulse.

3. Obstruction of the Channels and Collaterals by Trauma

With obvious traumatic history, drastic pain in the waist and lower extremities with activity disturbance, obvious local tenderness, ecchymoses on the tongue with thin whitish coating, taut and uneven pulse.

Treatment by Traditional Acupuncture

1. Body acupuncture

Prescription　**Dàchángshū(BL25)**, **Shènshū(BL23)**, **Huatuojiaji** point on the lumbar region, **Cìliáo (BL32)**, **Wěizhōng(BL40)**, **Yánglíngquán (GB34)** and **Xuánzhōng (GB39)**.

Supplementary points　For wind － cold － damp arthralgia, **Dàzhuī(DU14)** and **Yīnlíngquán(SP9)** are added; for deficiency of the kidney － essence, **Pángguāngshū (BL28)** and **Tàixī (KI3)**; for blood stasis obstructing collaterals, **Shuǐgōu(DU26)** and points which reveal tenderness on palpation.

Method: Use filiform needles to puncture the points with reinforcing or even movement method.

2. Auricular acupuncture

Prescription　Zuogushenjing (AH_6) sciatic nerve, Tun (AH_7) gluteus, Yaodizhui (AH_9) lumbosacral vertebrae, Shenmen(TF_4) shenmen and Pizhixia(AT_4) subcortex.

Method　Select 2 － 3 points for each treatment. Give a moderate and strong stimulation to the points. Retain the needles for 30 minutes. Give the treatment once a day. The seed － embedding therapy is also applicable.

3. Eletrotherapy

Prescription　**Jiaji (EX － B2)** on the lumbar region,

Yánglíngquán(GB34) and Wěizhōng(BL40).

Method   Insert the needles into the points. After arrival of qi, electrify them for 20 minutes with a dense wave or a sparse – dense wave. Give the treatment once daily.

4. Hand Acupuncture

1) Wind and dampness type

The patients may suffer from pain and heaviness of lower limb radiated along foot Taiyang urinary bladder meridian, impairment of movement of joints, numbness of skin and paralysis of muslces. The tongue proper is pale with white and greasy coating and the pulse is soft and moderate.

Therapeutic principle   To expel wind, eliminate dampness and improve movement of joints.

Principal   acupoints   **Zuògǔshénjīngdiǎn**   and **Yāotòngdiǎn(EX – UE7)**.

Supplemental acupoints   **Xiǎochángdiǎn** and **Yángchí (SJ4)**.

The   moxibustion   with   aconite   is   applied   to **Zuògǔshénjīngdiǎn** with moxa cones in a size of a pit of date and changed for 5 times in patients with severe pain and spasm of lower limb, which may be exacerbated by coldness, cough or sneezing; the warm acupuncture is applied at **Yángchí(SJ4)**; and the moxibustion with ginger is applied to **Yāotòngdiǎn(EX – UE7)** with moxa cones changed for 3 times.

2) Damp – heat type   The patients may suffer from

burning pain and difficult movement of lower limb, fever and thirst. The tongue proper is red in color with yellow and greasy or yellow and dry coating and the pulse is rolling and rapid.

Therapeutic principle　To clear heat, eliminate dampness and release stasis is collaterals.

Principal acupoints　**Yángchí**(SJ4), and **Yāotòngdiǎn** (**EX－UE7**).

3) Deficiency of liver and kidney Yin

The patients may suffer from pain, spasm and rigidity of waist and leg, lightning sensation in leg during walking, muscular twitches during episode of pain, hotness in sole, difficulty to stand straight and dryness in mouth without desire to drink water. The tongue proper is red in color with thin or scanty coating and the pulse is wiry and thready.

Therapeutic principle　To tonify liver and kidney, relax muscles and improve movement of joints.

Principal acupoints　**Láogōng**(PC8) and **Hégǔ**(LI4).

Supplemental acupoints　**Huántiào**(GB30), **Shèndiǎn**.

Therapeutic Methods by Practising Qigong

1. Self Treatment by Practising Qigong

1) Basic Maneuvers

It is advisable to practise Waist Qigong and Lower Limbs Qigong.

2) Auxiliary Maneuvers

(1) Arthralgia due to wind – cold – dampness: It is advisable to practise Eight – Section Brocade and Six – Section Brocade.

(2) Deficiency of the liver and kidney: It is advisable to practise the method of strengthening the kidney and conducting qi in Regulating – Kidney Qigong as well as the method of soothing the liver and conducting qi in Regulating – Liver Qigong.

(3) Obstruction of the channels and collaterals by traumata: It is advisable to practise Conducting Qigong to raise and lower yin and yang.

2. External Qi Therapy

(1) Press and knead **Shènshū (BL23), Mìngmén (DU4), Yāoyángguān (DU3), Huántiào (GB30), Yánglíngquán (GB34), Wěizhōng (BL40), Chéngshān (BL57), Kūnlún(BL60) and Tàixī(KI3)**.

(2) Deficiency of the Liver and Kidney

Apply the flat – palm form, use the pulling and rotating manipulations to emit qi onto **Shènshū (BL23), Mìngmén (DU4)**, and conduct the channel qi along the Urinary Bladder Meridian to the lower limbs.

(3) Apply flat – palm form, use the pushing, pulling, and leading manipulations to emit qi onto **Huántiào(GB30)** and conduct qi to the lower limbs so as to make qi balanced.

2) Auxiliary Maneuvers

(1) Arthralgia − syndrome due to wind − cold − dampness   Add the heatstyle conducting − qi method, apply the flat − palm form, use the pulling and leading manipulations to pull the pathogenic qi along the channel out of the body.

(2) Deficiency of the liver and kidney   Apply the flat − palm form, use pulling and rotating manipulations to emit qi onto **Shènshū** (**BL**23), **Mìngmén** (**DU**4) and **Guānyuán** (**RN**4).

(3) Obstruction of the channels and collaterals by trauma   Apply flat − palm form, use rotating and leading manipulations to conduct the channel qi along the channels and make use of the wrenching and rocking manipulations.

Therapeutic Methods by Chinese Massage

Massage therapy of this disease may produce obvious curative effect in most cases. A secondary case should be treated comprehensively by integrating with the manipulation of massage for the primary case. In addition, a careful differential diagnosis is needed and the massage therapy is forbidden in sciatica caused by tumor, metastatic carcinoma, tuberculosis, etc. .

1. Manipulation   Digital − pressing, pressing, kneading, rolling and traction.

2. Points Selection   **Dàchángshū** (**BL**25), **Zhìbiān** (**BL**54), **Huántiào** (**GB**30), **Chéngfú** (**BL**36), **Yīnmén** (**BL**37), **Liángqiū** (**ST**34), **Yánglíngquán** (**GB**34),

Chéngshān(BL57), Jiěxī(ST41), Kūnlún(BL60).

3. Operation

1) The doctor stands at the affected side of the patient who is in prone position and then applies rolling manipulation for 3 to 5 times to the lumbar muscle of the affected side of the lower lumbar vertebrae and along the posterior aspect of the affected thigh and the posterolateral part of the leg softly at first and then hard and deeply.

2) Then the doctor, with the thumbs overlapped press – kneads the points revealed pain on the waist and the buttock for one two minutes repeatedly with a bit more strength.

3) Using his elbow, the doctor presses the points of **Dàchángshū(BL25)** and **Huántiào(GB30)** and the points revealed pain on the waist and the buttock.

4) The doctor digit – presses the points of **Chéngfú (BL36), Yīnmén(BL37), Wěizhōng(BL40), Chéngshān (BL57), Kūnlún(BL60)**, etc..

5) The doctor holds the lumbus and pulls it backwards, once for the right and once for the left.

6) Repeat Operation 1) twice to 3 times.

7) The patient is in prone position, while the doctor, digit – presses to stimulate the points of **Fútù (ST32), Liángqiū(ST34), Zúsānlǐ(ST36), Yánglíngquán(GB34), Xuánzhōng** and **Jiěxī(ST41)**. Then the doctor rolls from the upper part to the lower part and repeats the operation twice

to 3 times.

8) Ask the patient to flex his knee and hip bone. Then the doctor, with one hand grasping the foot sole, the other supporting the affected knee, makes the patient do compulsory flexion of the hip bone, stretch the knee and extend the ankle, twice to 3 times. Be sure that the stretching angle of the lower limb should be within the limits of the patient's movement.

9) Let the patient's lower limb stretch straight and accomplish the operation with the manipulation of foulaging and shaking the lower limb.

4. Course of Treatment   Once a day, 10 days for one course with an interval of 5 − 7 days between two courses.

Polyneuritis

Polyneuritis, also called peripheral neuritis, is usually caused by infection, allergy, intoxication and metabolic disturbance. Therefore, the patients may develop symmetrical sensory impairment of distal part of 4 limbs, flaccid paralysis, disturbance of vegetative nervous system and nutritive and functional disorders.

Etiology and Pathogenesis

The etiological factors can be divided into external and internal varieties. The external pathogenic factors contain the epidemic heat pathogens to cause influenza, typhoid and mumps. The heat pathogens retained in body may cause lower fever, injury of lungs scorched by heat, consumption of body fluid and loss of fluid to supply the muscles and blood vessels. The retention of external dampness pathogen may produce heat and the damp – heat pathogen may block circulation of qi and blood and injure muscles and blood vessels to cause numbness of skin and paralysis of muscles. The internal pathogenic factors contain the metabolic, endocrinal and nutritive disturbances. The deficiency and weakness of spleen may imperil the digestive function, so that the spleen can not produce enough qi, blood and body fluid to nourish muscles and blood vessels. The liver can store blood and control tendons and the kidney can store essence and control bones. Therefore, the muscles and blood vessels may lose nutrients and fluid and the limbs may lose their locomotive function, if the liver and kidney are deficient. At the early stage, the patients have pain and numbness of limbs, so that the disease is belonged to the Bi – syndrome in traditional Chinese medicine; and at the late stage, the patients have impairment of sensory and locomotive function and muscular atrophy, therefore, it is belonged to the Wei – syndrome (paralytic disease).

Differential Diagnosis and Treatment

1) Damp – heat type

The patients may suffer from numbness, heaviness, weakness, pain and formication of limbs, worse in lower limbs and in distal ends of the limbs. The loss of sensation of limbs may show a glove or sock pattern in distribution and then the region of sensory disturbance may gradually spread to the proximal ends of limbs. The patients may also suffer from lower fever or tidal fever, chest distress and short stream of dark urine. The tongue proper is red in color with yellow and greasy coating and the pulse is soft and rapid.

Therapeutic principle　　To clear heat and eliminate dampness.

Principal acupoint　**Bāxié(EX – UE9)**.

Supplemental acupoints　**Yángchí(SJ4)**, **Shèndiǎn**.

The bleeding therapy is applied at **Bāxié(EX – UE9)**; and Dadun (LR 1), **Yújì(LU10)** and **Láogōng(PC8)** may be used in patients with much heat pathogen.

2) Cold and dampness type

The patients may suffer from pain of limbs, hatred of coldness, muscular atrophy, profuse sweating or no sweat, foot drop, reduction of food intake and loose stool. The tongue proper is pale with thin and white coating and the pulse is slow.

Therapeutic principle　　To warm meridians, eliminate dampness and expel cold pathogen.

Principal acupoint　**Sānjiāodiǎn**.

Supplemental acupoints　**Hégǔ(LI4)**, **Yángchí(SJ4)**, **Shèndiǎn**.

The warm acupuncture may be applied at **Sānjiāodiǎn**, **Yángchí(SJ4)** and **Shēnmài(BL62)**.

3) Deficiency of liver and kidney　　The patients may suffer from numbness and spasm of distal ends of limbs, foot

drop, muscular atrophy of lower limbs, soreness and weakness of spinal column and waist, vertigo, tinnitus, dryness in mouth without desire to drink water and dark urine. The tongue proper is red in color with yellow or scanty coating and the pulse is thready and rapid.

Therapeutic principle　To tonify liver and kidney, enrich Yin and clear heat.

Principal acupoints　**Shèndiǎn** and **Láogōng(PC8)**.

Supplemental acupoints　**Yújì（LU10）**, **Nèiguān (PC6)**, **Gāndiǎn**, **Sānjiāodiǎn**.

Rheumatic Arthritis

Rheumatic arthritis is a systemic collagen disease with repeated attacks of arthralgia as an allergic disease caused by infection of hemolytic streptococcus. It is belonged to Bi – syndrome in traditional Chinese medicine.

Etiology and Pathogenesis

Rheumatic arthritis is caused by invasion of wind, cold, dampness and heat pathogens into meridians to block circulation of qi, blood and Yang qi. The pathogens in meridians may migrate up and down to produce wandering pain radiated all over the body. It is called Zhou (throughout) Bi – syndrome in traditional Chinese medicine.

Differential Diagnosis and Treatment

1) Wind and damp – heat type

The patients may suffer from sour or distending pain in the joints of whole body, headache, fever, nodules and annular erythema on both lower limbs, wandering arthralgia and dryness in mouth without desire to drink water. The tongue proper is red in color with thin and white coating and the pulse is rapid or rolling and rapid.

Therapeutic principle   To disperse wind, eliminate dampness and clear heat.

Principal acupoints   **Bāxié (EX – UE9), Gāndiǎn, Hégǔ(LI4).**

Supplemental acupoints   **Yāotòngdiǎn (EX – UE7), Zuògǔshénjīngdiǎn, Jǐzhùdiǎn.**

'   2) Cold and dampness type   The patients may suffer from swelling and severe fixed pain of joints worsened by coldness and improved by hotness. The tongue proper is pale with thin and white coating and the pulse is deep and tense or wiry and tense.

Therapeutic principle   To expel cold, warm meridians and eliminate dampness.

Principal acupoints   **Hégǔ(LI4), Yángchí(SJ4)** and **Shèndiǎn.**

Supplemental acupoints   **Sānjiāodiǎn** and **Yāotòngdiǎn (EX – UE7).**

Edema

Edema is a common symptom appeared in many diseases with swelling of face, head, limbs, abdomen and even whole body due to accumulation of water in the skin and muscles.

Etiology and Pathogenesis

The invasion of wind pathogen to the body surface may inhibit the function of lungs to disperse qi and downward transport water to urinary bladder. The water conjugated with wind pathogen may be distributed and retained in skin and muscles to produce edema. The external dampness pathogen may invade the spleen and imperil the digestive function of spleen to cause accumulation of water in the body to produce edema.

Differential Diagnosis and Treatment

1) Yang type of edema

The edema may appear on the face and head first and spread to whole body, but more prominent above the waist. The skin is bright and the edema of skin is pitting in nature. The patients may also suffer from oliguria, chillness, fever, soreness and pain of limbs, cough with rough breath sound. The patients caused by wind and cold pathogen may have cold limbs without sweating, the tongue coating is white and slippery and the pulse is floating and tense; the patients caused by wind and heat pathogen may have sore throat, the tongue coating is thin and yellow and the pulse is floating and rapid.

Therapeutic principle   To disperse wind and lung qi, promote discharge of water and resolve swelling.

Principal acupoints   **Fèidiǎn** and **Pídiǎn**.

Supplemental acupoints   **Dàchángdiǎn** and **Xiàngǔ** (**ST**43). The reducing technique is used to apply acupuncture; the moxibustion is used to treat patients caused by wind and cold pathogens; and pricking therapy is applied to patients caused by wind and heat pathogens.

2) Yin type of edema

The edema first appears on the feet and gradually spread

upward, but more remarkable below waist. The skin is dark and the edema is pitting in nature. The patients may also suffer from oliguria, distension of upper abdomen, diarrhea with loose stool and tiredness of limbs. In patients with deficiency of spleen, the tongue coating is white and greasy and the pulse is soft and moderate; and the patients with deficiency of kidney may suffer from soreness and weakness of waist and legs, cold limbs and mental tiredness, the tongue proper is pale with white coating and the pulse is deep, thready and weak.

Therapeutic principle   To strengthen spleen, warm kidney, enrich Yang and promote the discharge of water.

Principal acupoints   **Shèndiǎn** and **Pídiǎn**.

The balanced reinforce − reducing technique is used to apply acupuncture and the moxibustion may be used in combination for Yin type of edema. More reducing technique is applied to physically stronger patients; and more reinforcing technique with moxibustion is applied to weaker patients.

Diabetes Mellitus

Clinical diabetes mellitus represents a syndrome with disordered metabolism and inappropriate hyperglycemia due to either an absolute deficiency of insulin secretion or a reduction in its biologic effectiveness or both and leading to metabolic disturbance of carbohydrate, fat and protein. The disease is frequently followed by water − electrolyte imbalance and acid − base disturbance. According to the age of the patients, clinical manifestation and requirements for insulin, diabetes mellitus can be divided into many types.

The national institutes of health in 1979 decided to defer a "functional" classification of diabetes that based upon insulin secretion characteristics of insulin sensitivity. It recommends classifying diabetes mellitus into 2 major types.

Type I   Insulin − Dependent Diabetes Mellitus (ID-DM). This severe form is associated with ketosis in the untreated state. It occurs most commonly in juveniles but also occasionally in adults.

Type Ⅱ   Non − Insulin − Dependent Diabetes Mellitus (NIDDM). This represents a heterogeneous group comprising milder forms of diabetes that occur predominantly in adults but occasionally in juveniles. Two subgroups of patients with Type II diabetes are currently distinguished by the absence or presence of obesity.

a. Nonobese NIDDM patients   These patients generally show an absent or blunted early phase of insulin release in response to glucose.

b. Obese NIDDM patients   This form of diabetes is secondary to extrapancreatic factors that produce insensitivity to endogenous insulin.

In traditional Chinese medicine, the modern term for the condition is "emaciation − thirst disease". But in ancient Chinese medicine, it is called "Shi Yi" or "Xiao Dan". The diagnosis is mainly based on symptoms such as thirst, polydipsia, polyphagia, emaciation and polyuria.

Etiology and Pathogenesis

Diabetes occurs in association with the following etiologic factors:

1. The spleen and stomach are damaged by overeating greasy food or by overconsuming alcohol causing failure of the spleen in transporting and transforming, which, in turn,

causes interior – heat to accumulate and consume food and body fluids, finally resulting in diabetes.

2. Impairment of body fluid

Deficiency of Yin and over – intake of rich fatty food and liquor contribute to accumulation of heat in the interior. The accumulated heat tends to turn to dryness. The dryness will impair body fluid.

3. Anxiety, anger and mental depression injure the liver, causing liver qi to stagnate. Protractedly stagnated liver qi turn into pathogenic heat which consumes body fluids and eventually leads to diabetes.

4. Deficiency in the kidneys caused by intemperance in sexual life or congenital essence defect causes kidney qi to wane; as a result, kidney qi fails to maintain the function of the bladder in restraining urine discharge, thus polyuria occurs.

5. Burned Yin – fluid of the lung and stomach

long – term of emotional stimulus leads to stagnation of Qi. Stagnation of Qi leads to production of fire . The fire burns Yin – fluid of the lung and stomach.

6. Attack of the lung and stomach by hyperactive fire

Overstrain and sexual intemperance exhaust Yin – essence. Exhaustion of Yin – essence causes deficiency of Yin. Yin – deficiency results in hyperactivity of fire. The resulting fire will go upward to heat the lung and stomach.

Main Symptoms and Signs

The classic symptoms of polyuria, thirst, recurrent blurred vision, paresthesias and fatigue are manifestations of hyperglycemia and thus are common to both major types of diabetes , likewise, pruritus vulvae and vaginitis are frequent initial complaints of adult females with hyperglycemia and glycosuria due to either absolute or relative deficiencies of insulin. Weight loss despite normal or increased appetite is a feature of IDDM, whereas weight loss is unusual in obese patients with NIDDM who have normal or increased levels of circulating insulin. These latter patients with the insulin − insensitive type of diabetes may be relatively asymptomatic and may be detected only after glycosuria or hyperglycemia is noted during a routine examination. Diabetes should be suspected in obese patients, in those with a positive family history of diabetes, in patients presenting with peripheral neuropathy and in women who have delivered large babies or had polyhydramnios, preeclampsia, or unexplained fetal losses.

Main Points of Diagnosis

1. The characteristics of a typical case of diabetes mellitus are often polyphagia, polydipsia, polyuria and loss of body weight. Early or asymptomatic patients only show ab-

normal release of cortical hormone and insulin inside the body. The level of fasting blood sugar is elevated with abnormal glucose tolerance test. Symptomatic patients are frequently complicated by other symptoms of dermal, neural and endocrinous disorders in addition to polyphogia, polydipsia, polyuria and emaciation.

2. The main complications and concomitant diseases of diabetes mellitus are diabetic ketoacidosis , cardiovascular diseases, diabetic renopathy and peripheral neuropathy. Cardiovascular complications are the chief causes of death.

3. Diabetes mellitus is classified into juvenile and adult types according to the clinical features. The age of onset of the juvenile type is young and has a tendency to inheritance. Blood sugar fluctuates widely and is quite sensitive to insulin. Treatment is difficult and is easily complicated by ketoacidosis and hypoglycemia, and so it is often named insulin − depending diabetes or unstable diabetes. The age of onset of adult type is above 40. This type is relatively mild and can be controlled by dietary restriction or oral antidiabetics. Therefore it is also named non − insulin depending diabetes or stable diabetes.

4. Accessory examination

(1) Fasting blood − glucose is higher than 130 − 140 mg/dl. Blood glucose after meal is more than 160 − 180 mg/dl. Urine is positive for glucose. If complicated by ketosis, urine is positive for ketone bodies.

(2) Fasting plasma glucose is less than 140 mg/dl in suspected cases. A standardized oral glucose tolerance test may be done. Glucose tolerance test can be used to diagnose early or suspected cases and is the principal test in diagnosis.

The National Diabetes Data Group recommends giving a 75g glucose dose dissolved in 300ml of water for adults (1.75 per kg ideal body weight for children) after an over – night fast in subjects who have been receiving at least 150 – 200g of carbohydrate daily for 3 days before the test.

Normal glucose tolerance is considered to be present when the 2 – hour plasma glucose is less than 140 mg/dl, with no value between zero time and 2 hours exceeding 200 mg/dl. However, a diagnosis of diabetes mellitus requires plasma glucose levels to be 200 mg/dl both at 2 hours and at least twice between zero time and 2 hours.

(3) New diagnostic techniques such as testing blood insulin levels are quite helpful in understanding the pathological changes of pancreas and in obtaining information concerning treatment.

(4) Insulin levels during glucose tolerance test. Normal immunoreactive insulin levels range from less than 10 to 25 $\mu V/ml$ in the fasting state and 50 to 130 $\mu V/ml$ at 1 hour and usually return to levels below $100\mu V/ml$ by 2 hours. A value below $50\mu V/ml$ at 1 hour and less than $100\mu V/ml$ at 2 hours in the presence of sustained hyperglycemia implicates insensitivity of B cells to glucose as the cause of hyperglyce-

mia, whereas levels substantially above $100\mu V/ml$ at these times suggest tissue unresponsiveness to the action of insulin.

Diet:

Caloric restriction for obese patients and regular spaced feeding with a bedtime snack for patients receiving hypoglycemic agents, especially insulin.

A well – balanced nutritious diet remains a fundamental element of therapy. However, in more than half of cases, diabetic patients fail to follow their diet. The reasons for this are varied and include unnecessary complexity of the prescription as well as lack of understanding of the goals by both the patient and the physician. In prescribing a diet, it is important to relate dietary objectives to the type of diabetes. In obese patients with mild hyperglycemia, the major goal of diet therapy is weight reduction by caloric restriction. Thus, there is less need for exchange lists. Emphasis on timing of meals, or periodic snacks, all of which are so essential in the treatment of insulin requiring nonobese diabetics.

Because of the prevalence of the obese mild diabetic among the population of diabetics receiving therapy, this type of patient represents the most frequent and this one of the most important challenges for the physician. Treatment requires an energetic, vigorous program directed by persons who are aware of the mechanisms by which weight reduction is known to effectively lower hyperglycemia and who are convinced of the profoundly beneficial effects of weight control on blood lipid levels as well as on hyperglycemia in obese diabetics. Weight reduction is an elusive goal that can only be achieved by close supervision of the obese patient.

Ⅱ. The traditional classification of "xiao ke" – – four traditional types in traditional Chinese medicine

In traditional Chinese medicine, the condition is divided into four types: emaciation – polydipsia of the upper part of the body, emaciation – polydipsia of the middle part of the body, emaciation – polydipsia of the lower part of the body and stagnant blood and Qi.

Differential Diagnosis and Treatment

Upper type of diabetes

The patients may suffer from extreme thirst with desire to drink much water, dryness in mouth and throat, occasional diuresis and overeating. The tongue tip is red, the coating is yellow and thin and the pulse is full and rapid.

Therapeutic principle   To clear lung heat, moisten dryness, produce saliva and relieve thirst.

Principal acupoints **Fèidiǎn** and **Pídiǎn**.

Supplemental acupoints   **Wèichángtòngdiǎn** and **Shèndiǎn**.

2) Middle type of diabetes

The patients may have severe hunger and desire to eat much food, distress in stomach, hot feeling in body and annoyance, profuse sweating, pathological leanness, constipation and occasional diuresis and drinking much water. The tongue coating is yellow and dry and the pulse is rolling and rapid.

Therapeutic principle　To clear stomach fire, tonify Yin and produce saliva.

Principal acupoints　**Shàofǔ(HT8)** and **Sānjiāodiǎn**.

Supplemental acupoints　**Pángguāngshū(BL28)**, **Píshū (BL20)**.

3) Lower type of diabetes

The patients may suffer from frequent urinatioin of a large amount of sticky urine, dryness in mouth and tongue, thirst with desire to drink much water, dizziness, vertigo, flushed cheeks, annoyance, soreness and weakness of wait and knee. The tongue is red in color and the pulse is thready and rapid. The chronic patients with deficiency of both Yin and Yang may have cold body and limbs and profuse discharge of urine. The tongue proper is pale with white coating and the pulse is deep, thready and weak.

Therapeutic principle　To tonify kidney Yin.

Principal acupoints　**Shèndiǎn** and **Yángchí(SJ4)**.

Supplemental acupoints　**Láogōng(PC8)**, **Hégǔ(LI4)** and **Shàoshāng(LU11)**.

The diabetes mellitus is a disease with clinical manifestation of excessive symptoms, although it is caused by deficient pathogenic factors, so that it should be treated with the balanced reinforce − reducing technique of acupuncture. In chronic patients the moxibustion may be used in combination, once a day or every 2 days. The treatment should be continued for a period of time to maintain the therapeutic effect after the clinical symptoms are relieved.

The acupuncture can produce certain therapeutic effect in patients of mild and moderate severity, but it is less effective in insulin − dependent cases or patients at late stage. Therefore, the early diagnosis and early treatment of this disease is very important. Because the diabetic patients are very weak and susceptible to infection, the rules of sterilization for application of acupuncture should be strictly followed. The diabetic patients with acidosis may suffer from nausea, vomiting, abdominal pain, dyspnea, drowsiness and even coma, hypotension and circulatory failure. The breath is deep and quick with a smell of rotten apple. The patients with ketoacidosis should be effectively rescued in time with a combined therapy of traditional and western medicine.

The diabetic patients should be on a rational dietary regimen with food rich in protein and vegetables and limited carbohydrates. They should also carry on an adequate physical exercise to strengthen their body.

Incontinence of Urine

Incontinence of urine is a symptom with spontaneous discharge of urine out of voluntary control and loss of sense of urination.

Etiology and Pathogenesis

The incontinence of urine is caused by dysfunction of urinary bladder, but it is also related to lung, spleen and kidney organs. The important function of kidney is to store essence and restrict the discharge of urine under voluntary control. The urinary bladder may fail to control the regular discharge of urine, if the kidney is deficient and can not store essence. The deficiency of spleen and stomach qi may cause impairment of their digestive and transporting function. It may also disturb the function of urinary bladder to control the discharge of urine. The heart is a fire organ to control mental activity and the kidney is a water organ to store

essence. Therefore, when the heart fire can not warm the
kidney water and the heart and kidney can not mutually
communicate, the incontinence of urine may happen.

Differential Diagnosis and Treatment

1) Deficiency of spleen and kidney

The urine may be spontaneously discharged out of voluntary control and the patients may suffer from low spirit,
weakness of limbs, fear of coldness and soreness and weakness of waist and knee. The tongue is pale with thin and
white coating and the pulse is deep, thready and weak.

Therapeutic principle   To tonify spleen and kidney.

Principal acupoints   **Láogōng(PC8)** and **Sānjiāodiǎn**.

Supplemental acupoints   **Pángguāngshū(BL28)**, and
Shèndiǎn.

The moxibustion with aconite is applied to
Pángguāngshū(BL28) with moxa cones in a size of a wheat
grain and changed for 5 times.

2) Deficiency of qi and blood

The discharge of urine is out of voluntary control after
external trauma and the patients may also suffer from sallow
complexion and distending sensation and discomfort of waist.
The tongue proper is dark purple with petechiae, the tongue
coating is thin and white and the pulse is wiry and thready.

Therapeutic principle   To adjust qi and regulate the

function of urinary bladder.

Principal acupoints **Sānjiāodiǎn** and **Shèndiǎn**.

Supplemental acupoints **Zhōngjí(RN3)**, **Xīndiǎn**.

The warm acupuncture is applied at **Sānjiāodiǎn** and **Shèndiǎn**.

Retention of Urine

Retention of urine is a symptom with urine retained in the urinary bladder and incapably discharged voluntarily out of the body.

Etiology and Pathogenesis

The pathogenic organ of this symptom is the urinary bladder. However, the formation and discharge of urine is also closely related to Sanjiao (triple energizer). If the upper energizer can not adjust transmission of body fluid all over the body, including the urinary bladder; the middle energizer can not separate the clear and turbid fluid; and the lower energizer can not filter and drain the waste fluid out of body, then the urine may be retained in the urinary bladder and can not be discharged from the body. The kidney is a storage organ and can control the orifices for discharge of urine and stool. If the function of kidney to control those orifices is disturbed, the urine will be retained in the urinary bladder. The retention of urine may also be caused by accumulation of damp – heat and other turbid pathogen in body, blockage of Yang qi by invaded cold and dampness pathogen, external trauma with stagnation of qi and blood as well as obstruction of urinary tract by renal stones or after surgical operations.

Differential Diagnosis and Treatment

1) Damp – heat type

The patients may suffer from retention of urine and discharge of urine by drops, distension of lower abdomen, bitter taste and sticky sensation in mouth or thirst without desire to drink water, annoyance, nausea and vomiting. The tongue proper is red in color with yellow and greasy coating and the pulse is wiry and rapid or soft and rapid.

Therapeutic principle   To clear heat and eliminate dampness.

Principal acupoints   **Sānjiāodiǎn** and **Shèndiǎn**.

Supplemental acupoints   **Guānyuán** (RN4), **Zhōngjí** (RN3), **Pángguāngshū**(BL28), **Sānjiāoshū**(BL22).

2) Cold and dampness type

The patients may also suffer from fear of coldnes, cold limbs, dark complexion, regurgitation of clear water, poor appetite, no desire to speak and move and shortness of breath. The tongue coating is pale with white and greasy coating. The pulse is deep and thready and the pulse at Chi position is weak.

Therapeutic principle   To warm kidney, strengthen spleen, eliminate dampness and promote discharge of water.

Principal acupoints   **Mìngméndiǎn** and **Sānjiāodiǎn**.

Supplemental acupoints   **Shèndiǎn, Guānyuán(RN4), Sānjiāoshū(BL22)**. The moxibustion with aconite is applied to **Guānyuán(RN4)** with moxa cones changed for 3 times until the local skin is flushed; and the paste of single clove garlic is applied over **Guānyuán(RN4)**.

3) Stagnation of qi type

The patients may suffer from retention of urine, straining and distension of lower abdomen, pain and distension of flank and costal region, anorexia, nausea and vomiting. The tongue proper is pale with thin and white coating and the pulse is wiry.

Therapeutic principle   To disperse liver qi and promote the discharge of urine.

Principal acupoints   **Zhōngjí(RN3)** and **Shèndiǎn**.

Supplemental acupoints   **Pángguāngshū (BL28), Sānjiāodiǎn**.

4) Deficiency of qi type: The patients may suffer from pale complexion, shortness of breath, dyspnea, spontaneous sweating, weakness, poor appetite and difficulty to pass urine although with desire of urination. The tongue proper is pale with thin and white coating and the pulse is deep and

weak.

　　Therapeutic principle　To tonify spleen qi.

　　Principal acupoints　**Pídiǎn** and **Mìngméndiǎn**.

　　Supplemental acupoints　**Shèndiǎn, Píshū**(**BL20**) and **Fèidiǎn**. The warm acupuncture is applied to **Píshū**(**BL20**).

5) External trauma type

　　After external trauma or surgical operation, the patients may suffer from difficulty to pass urine with distended urinary bladder and annoyance. The tongue proper is red in color with thin and white coating and the pulse is deep and wiry.

　　Therapeutic principle　To promote circulation of qi and blood and promote discharge of urine.

　　Principal acupoint　**Guānyuán**(**RN4**).

　　Supplemental acupoints　**Shèndiǎn, Pángguāngshū**(**BL28**), **Sānjiāodiǎn**.

　　The finger－pressing massage may be applied at a spot 2.5 cun below umbilicus with pressure gradually increased until the urine is discharged.

Impotence

Impotence is a symptom with penis failed to firmly erect for sexual intercourse.

Etiology and Pathogenesis

The kidney can store essence and its external orifices are the anus and meatus of urethra. The liver can store blood and its meridian passes around the external genitalia. The Yangming meridian controls the penis. Before adolescence, the kidney qi is still insufficient, so that the early marriage and masturbation may deplete the kidney qi. In adults the congenital deficiency of essence, indulgence of sexual activity and poor rehabilitation of disease may cause deficiency of kidney Yang to produce impotence. The worriment can cause impotence because it may damage heart and spleen to interfere the intake of food and formation of blood and essence to supply the penis. The impotence may also be caused by de-

pletion of kidney qi due to frightening or by injury of liver
and kidney due to accumulation of damp − heat in Yangming
meridian and transmission of this pathogen to liver and kidney.

Differential Diagnosis and Treatment

1) Deficiency of kidney Yang

The patients may suffer from impotence, pale complexion, soreness and weakness of waist and leg and vertigo. The
tongue proper is pale with thin and white coating and the
pulse is deep and thready.

Therapeutic principle   To warm kidney and tonify
Yang.

Principal acupoints   **Guānyuán(RN4)** and **Shèndiǎn**.

Supplemental acupoints   **Sānjiāodiǎn** and **Sānjiāoshū**
(**BL**22). The moxibustion with aconite is applied to
Sānjiāodiǎn and **Sānjiāoshū**(**BL**22) with moxa cones in a
size of a pit of date and changed for 3 times.

2) Deficiency of heart and spleen

The patients may suffer from impotence, sallow complexion, physical and mental tiredness, insomnia and poor
appetite. The tongue proper is pale with white coating and
the pulse is thready and weak.

Therapeutic principle   To tonify heart and spleen.

Principal acupoints   **Xīndiǎn** and **Pídiǎn**.

Supplemental acupoints   **Xīnshū (BL15)**, **Píshū (BL20)**, **Sānjiāodiǎn**.

3) Downward flowing of damp – heat

The patients may suffer from impotence, heaviness of lower limbs, cold sweating and dark hot urine. The tongue proper is red in color with yellow and greasy coating and the pulse is soft and rapid.

Therapeutic principle   To clear damp – heat.

Principal acupoints   **Láogōng (PC8)** and **Shàoshāng (LU11)**.

Supplemental acupoints   **Guānyuán (RN4)**, **Sānjiāodiǎn** and **Pídiǎn**.

Emission of Semen

Emission of semen is a symptom of spontaneous ejaculation of semen without sexual coitus. It can be divided into 2 types: with or without dream of sexual behavior. The pathogenesis and treatment of both types are the same.

Etiology and Pathogenesis

The pathogenic organs of emission are heart, liver and kidney. The heart is an organ with monarch fire (heart fire) to administer mental activity; and the kidney is an organ with ministerial fire (kidney fire) to store essence. The liver and kidney are a pair of closely related organs and the essence in kidney and blood in liver can mutually transform. The indulgence in sexual life or frequent masturbation may cause deficiency of kidney qi and impairment of storage function of kidney due to exhaustion of kidney essence. The heart Yin can be wasted by mental overfatigue and the heart fire can be

exuberated after the heart Yin is depleted. If the heart fire
can not be balanced by kidney water and the water and fire
fail to balance each other, the communication between heart
and kidney may be interrupted. The monarch fire of heart
and ministerial fire of kidney may combine together to imperil the function of kidney to store semen and to disturb the
house of semen (seminal vesicle) to spontaneously discharge
the semen. The overeating of greasy and spicy food and alcohol may produce much damp – heat pathogen to stimulate the
house of semen to involuntarily discharge semen.

Differential Diagnosis and Treatment

1) Exacerbation of monarche and ministerial fire: The
patients may suffer from unstable sleep and emission with
dream, dizziness after emission, palpitation of heart, spiritlessness, tiredness and short stream of dark urine. The
tongue proper is red with thin and yellow coating and the
pulse is wiry and rapid.

Therapeutic principle   To clear fire of heart and kidney
and to arrest emission.

Principal acupoint   **Xīndiǎn, Shèndiǎn, Guānyuán**
(**RN4**).

Supplemental acupoints   **Láogōng** (**PC8**), **Shàofǔ**
(**HT8**). The reinforcing technique is applied to **Guānyuán**
(**RN4**); the reducing technique is applied to Taichong and

Zulinqi; balanced reinforcing – reducing technique is applied to **Xīndiǎn**; and the technique of fighting between dragon and tiger is applied to **Shèndiǎn**. The decoction of Lianzixin (lotus plumule) 9 gm, Huangbo (phellodendron bark) 10 gm, Rougui (cinnamon bark) 3 gm and Longgu (fossil bone) 20 gm may be orally administered, one dose per day.

2) Failure to store semen by deficient kidney   The patients may suffer from emission, dizziness, vertigo, tinnitus, soreness of waist, mental and physical tiredness. The tongue proper is red with scanty coating and the pulse is thready and rapid; or the coating is thin and yellow and the pulse at chi position is thready and weak.

Therapeutic principle   To tonify kidney Yin and arrest discharge of semen.

Principal acupoints   **Mìngméndiǎn** and **Shèndiǎn**.

Supplemental acupoints   **Shènshū (BL23)**, **Guānyuán (RN4)**, **Xīndiǎn**.

The respiratory reinforce – reducing technique is applied to **Shèndiǎn**; and the balanced reinforce – reducing technique is applied to **Guānyuán(RN4)** and **Xīndiǎn**.

3) Downward flowing of damp – heat pathogen   The patients may suffer from emission with dreams, white mucus in urine, bitter taste in mouth and thirst without desire to drink much water. The tongue proper is red in color with yellow coating and the pulse is soft and rapid.

Therapeutic principle   To clear heat, eliminate dampness and arrest emission of semen.

Principal acupoints   **Xīndiǎn** and **Láogōng(PC8)**.

Supplemental acupoints   **Shàofǔ(HT8)**, **Sānjiāodiǎn**, **Pídiǎn**. The reducing technique is applied to **Pídiǎn** and **Sānjiāodiǎn**; the reinforcing technique is applied to Taixi; and the balanced reinforce − reducing technique is applied to **Shàofǔ(HT8)**.

Chronic Prostatitis

Chronic prostatitis is a very common disease of the urinary system in the young and middle – aged male patients. The disease is usually a secondary infection of acute prostatitis or posterior urethritis. Sometimes, it may also be a secondary infection of the upper respiratory tract or mouth cavity. The common pathogens are *staphylococcus*, *streptococcus*, *colibacillus*, etc.. It is often induced by excessive alcoholic drinking, injury of the perineum, excessive sexual intercourses. This disease falls into the categories of *Jīngzhuó* and *Láolín* in traditional Chinese medicine.

Etiology and Pathogenesis

The door of essence room is unlocked because of excessive sexual intercourse. Damp – heat takes the opportunity to occupy the room, forcing sperm to flow to the urinary bladder and leave the body along with urine. Then, there will re-

sult deficiency of the kidney – yin, hyperactivity of the ministerial fire, disturbance of essence room and retention of
fire, all of which get together to lead to stagnation of qi and
blood in the spermatic duct and cause this disease at last. If
the disease course is prolonged, the deficient yin will involve
yang. At this time, there will occur syndrome due to insufficiency of the kidney – yang.

Main Symptoms and Signs

White and turbid drip from the urethral meatus commonly seen at the end of urination or in the course of having
a bowel movement with one's strength, or white sticky secretion from the urethral meatus usually found after getting
up in the morning; frequent urination and burning urine and
stabbing and itching urethra existing in most cases; tenesmus
and distention and pain in the lower abdomen, lumbosacral
portion, perineum and testes; listlessness, acratia, dizziness,
insomnia, sexual hypoesthesia, spermatorrhea, prospermia,
impotence and hemospermia.

Main Points of Diagnosis

1. Symptoms
1) Urinary Symptoms: There is frequent and urgent
micturition, pain in micturition and an uncomfortable urina-

tion or a burning feeling in micturition. At the end of urination or in moving the bowels, there is some sticky liquid dripping from the urethra.

2) Pain: There is a dull or a distending pain in the perineum and inside the rectum. The pain may radiate to the lumbosacral portion, the hip, the thigh, the testicle, the groin, etc..

3) Disturbance of Sexual Function: It is marked by sexual hypoesthesia, impotence, prospermia, pain in ejaculation, hemospermia, nocturnal emission, etc..

4) Constitutional Symptoms: There are neurasthenic symptoms such as weakness and fatigue in the whole body, aching pain at the waist and the back, insomnia, dreaminess, etc.. Sometimes, diseases such as arthritis, endocarditis, iritis, conjunctivitis and peripheral neuritis may be initiated.

2. Examination

1) Rectal Examination: This examination elicits a swollen prostate with tumefaction and obvious tenderness. Sometimes, the prostate may be hard and smaller than the usual size. The surface may be uneven and feels as if here are nodes on it. But it can also be normal at times.

2) Examination of Prostatic Fluid: Massage the prostate to collect prostatic fluid and examine it through microscopy. In a serious case there will be a lot of pus cells and more than 10 white cells present in each high power field. On the other

hand, the lecithin corpuscles will obviously decrease or disappear.

3) The Three − glass Urine Test: If there are pus cells in the first glass and none in the second and the third glass or there are pus cells in the first and the third glass and none in the second that means the infection probably come from the prostate.

4) Bacterial Culture: After douching to sterilize and clean the urethra, massage prostate to collect the prostatic fluid for bacterial culture.

5) Use smear examination to find bacteria.

Differential Diagnosis and Treatment

1)Prostatitis of excess type

The patients may suffer from frequent, urgent and painful urination, terminal hematuria, straining and pain in perineal region radiated to lumbar and sacral region, external genitalia and thigh; or suffer from chillness, high fever, soreness and pain of whole body, headache, constipation and physical and mental tiredness; and the abscess of prostate gland may show fluctuation or perforation to drain pus into urethra, rectum or perineal region. The tongue proper is red in color with yellow and greasy coating and the pulse is rolling and rapid.

Therapeutic principle   To clear heat, remove toxic

pathogen and eliminate dampness.

Principal acupoints　**Shàoshāng**（LU11）,　**Láogōng**（PC8）.

Supplemental acupoints　**Pángguāngshū**（BL28）, **Shèndiǎn**. The bleeding therapy is applied to **Shíxuān**（EX－UE11）and **Shàoshāng**（LU11）to clear toxic－heat pathogen; the reducing technique is applied at **Shèndiǎn** with the needles retained for 30 min; and the balanced reinforce－reducing technique is applied to **Pángguāngshū**（BL28）. The decoction of honeysuckle flower 100 gm, phellodendron bark 20 gm, dandelion 30 gm, cogongrass rhizome 30 gm, talcum powder 30 gm and licorice root 5 gm may be drunk as tea. 2) Prostatitis of deficient type

The symptoms are not remarkable. The patients may suffer from dull pain in inguinal groove, mild pain of urination, dripping of urine after urination, burning sensation in urethra, discharge of white turbid fluid from urethra, or accompanied by impotence, emission of semen, annoyance and insomnia. The tongue proper is red with thin and white coating and the pulse is wiry.

Therapeutic principle　To eliminate dampness, release stasis in collaterals and tonify kidney.

Principal acupoints　**Láogōng**（PC8）, **Guānyuán**（RN4）and **Shèndiǎn**.

Supplemental acupoints　**Xīndiǎn**, **Sānjiāodiǎn**, **Xīnshū**（BL15）, **Shènshū**（BL23）.

The reducing technique is applied at **Xīndiǎn**; the balanced reinforce – reducing technique is applied to **Guānyuán**
(**RN4**); and the reinforcing technique is applied to
Shèndiǎn. The gentle moxibustion may be applied to above
acupoints for 30 min in patients with frequent urination,
soreness and weakness of waist and knee due to deficiency of
kidney Yang; the reinforcing technique may be applied to patients with deficiency of kidney Yin; the Zhibo Dihuang Pills
(a patent herbal drug) may be orally administered, 9 gm
tid.

Chapter Two
Skin and Surgical Diseases

Warts

Warts are the benign skin vegetations caused by virus infection and autoinoculation. In this group of skin diseases, there are the common warts, plantar warts, flat warts, infectious soft warts and pointed condyloma. All of them can be treated by foot acupuncture, except pointed condyloma.

Etiology and Pathogenesis

The liver can store blood and control tendons; and the spleen is in charge of digestion and it can control limbs and muscles. In patients with deficiency of liver and with dryness in blood, the tendons and blood vessels can not obtain enough nutrition; the invaded external wind and heat pathogens may be retained in skin and muscle to cause stagnation of qi and blood to produce the warts. The spleen is in charge of digestion and it can control limbs. In patients with deficiency of spleen, the excessive dampness pathogen may be accumulated to block circulation of qi to produce the warts.

Differential Diagnosis and Treatment

Clinical manifestation

The lesions of common warts are the papillary cornified skin vegetations in a size of a mung bean to a pea with a dry and rough surface, greyish brown or dirty yellow in color; the plantar warts on the toes and sole are tylotic in shape and yellow in color with scattered black spots; the flat warts are the scattered flat papules on the face and dorsum of hand with a smooth surface and in a light brown or normal skin color.

Therapeutic principle　　To expel pathogens, remove toxic pathogen, promote circulation of blood, release stasis of blood and suppress hyperactivity of liver.

Principal acupoints　**Shàofǔ(HT8)** and **Hégǔ(LI4)**.

Supplemental acupoints　**Bāxié(EX - UE9)**, and the center of primary wart (the first and biggest one).

The reducing technique is applied to above acupoints. The needle is inserted through the center of the primary wart to destroy the nutrient - supplying blood vessel, then the wart may shrink, wither and fall off.

After the local skin is sterilized, a moxa cone of the

same size as the wart is put on its top and lighted until the moxa is completely burned off with a pop sound audible. One moxa cone is enough. After the local skin is sterilized with 2.5% iodine tincture and 75% alcohal, the top of wart is punctured with a three – edged needle and some cheeselike substance may be squeezed out. Then the iodine tincture or phenol is applied to the wound.

Urticaria

Urticaria, or hives, is an allergic disease caused by contact with a specific precipitating factor (allergen). Some food, drugs, parasites, etc. can act as the allergens. It is marked by raised edematous patches of skin and mucous membrane and usually by intense itching. It is called "fēng zhěn kuài" in traditional Chinese medicine.

Etiology and Pathogenesis

The lungs are in charge of breath and they can control the skin and hair; and the spleen is in charge of digestion and it can control the limbs and muscles. In patients with poor defensive energy and reduced body resistance, the skin and muscles may be attacked by wind and heat pathogens to block the circulation of Yang qi and disturb the nutritive and protective function of body, so that the urticaria is produced. In patients with deficiency of spleen qi, the improper food may cause stagnation of food and accumulation of damp – heat, which may combine with the invaded wind pathogen to cause this disease. The change of living environment or insect bite may also cause urticaria.

Differential Diagnosis and Treatment

1) Stagnation of wind and cold pathogens

The skin lesions of pink urticaria of different size may fuse together to form large patches, distributed chiefly over the exposed part of body and they are induced by cold wind. The tongue coating is white in color and the pulse is soft or rolling.

Therapeutic principle   To expel wind and cold pathogen and adjust Ying (nutritive materials) and Wei (defensive energy) qi.

Principal acupoints   **Gāndiǎn, Bāxié(EX – UE9)**.

Supplemental acupoints   **Fèidiǎn, Láogōng(PC8)**.

The warm acupuncture is applied to **Mìngméndiǎn** for 30 min; and the reducing technique is applied to **Fèidiǎn**.

2) Stagnation of wind and heat pathogens

The skin lesions of urticaria are red, hot and like clouds with severe itching, worsened by hotness and relieved by coldness. The patients may also suffer from thirst, annoyance; or chillness, fever, sore throat; or stomachache, vomiting, abdominal pain and diarrhea. The tongue is red with

thin and white or light yellow coating and the pulse is floating and rapid.

Therapeutic principle   To disperse wind and clear heat
in skin and muscles.

Principal acupoint   **Bāxié(EX - UE9)**.

Supplemental acupoints   **Fèidiǎn** and **Pídiǎn**.

As the needle is removed, 1 ml of blood is bled from the
needling hole at **Bāxié(EX - UE9)** after the needle is retained for 30 min; the bleeding therapy is applied at
Shàoshāng(LU11); and the reducing technique is applied at
Fèidiǎn and **Pídiǎn**.

3) Damp - heat pathogen in spleen and stomach

The onset of the disease is prompt and the skin lesions
are red in color and fused together to form patches. The patients may also suffer from pain of upper abdomen, nausea,
vomiting, diarrhea with gurgling sound, soreness and pain of
knees and oligouria. The tongue proper is red with yellow
and greasy coating and the pulse is rolling and rapid.

Therapeutic principle   To tonify spleen and stomach,
expel wind and eliminate dampness pathogen.

Principal acupoints   **Shàoshāng(LU11)**, **Fèidiǎn**.

Supplemental acupoints   **Sānjiāodiǎn**, **Gāndiǎn**,
Pídiǎn.

The bleeding therapy is applied at **Shāngyáng(LI1)** and
Fèidiǎn; the reducing technique is applied to **Sānjiāodiǎn**,
Gāndiǎn and **Pídiǎn**.

The decoction of Huoxiang (giant – hyssop) 12 gm, Peilanye (eupatorium leaf) 10 gm and Lugen (reed rhizome) 30 gm is orally administered once a day.

4) Deficiency of heart and spleen

The skin lesions of pale papules induced by tiredness may repeatedly relapse and linger over a long period of time. The patients may also suffer from sallow complexion, physical and mental tiredness, palpitation of heart, shortness of breath and poor appetite. The tongue proper is pale with thin coating and the pulse is thready and weak.

Therapeutic principle   To tonify heart and spleen, remove pathogens from body surface and strengthen muscles.

Principal acupoints   **Pídiǎn** and **Xīndiǎn**.

Supplemental acupoints   **Píshū** (BL20), **Xīnshū** (**BL**15), **Sānjiāodiǎn**. The moxibustion with atractylodes is applied to **Xīndiǎn** and **Gāndiǎn**.

Erysipelas

Erysipelas is an acute febrile disease that is associated with intense often vesicular and edematous local inflammation of the skin and subcutaneous tissues and that is caused by a *hemolytic streptococcus*.

Etiology and Pathogenesis

The erysipelas is produced by the attack of fire and toxic heat pathogens to the skin to cause accumulation of qi and blood in meridians; after the invasion of wind, heat and damp – heat pathogens into the muscles, the toxic heat pathogen in blood may cause leakage of blood out of blood vessels to produce the skin lesion of erysipelas; and the toxic heat pathogen may further invade the internal organs to produce septicemia. Because the dampness is a turbid and sticky pathogen and difficult to eliminate, the erysipelas may repeatedly relapse. The accumulation of dampness in meridians of lower limbs over a long period of time may block the circulation of qi and blood to cause the elephantiasis of leg.

Differential Diagnosis and Treatment

Clinical manifestation

At the beginning, the patients may have chillness and high fever, general malaise, headache, thirst, vomiting and anorexia; and then the local small erythematous patch with clear elevated margins may appear with burning pain and the skin lesion with scattered small vesicles may gradually spread over bigger and bigger area. The patients may have swollen lower limb after repeated relapses and the urine is dark in color. The tongue proper is red with thin and yellow coating and the pulse is thready and rapid.

Therapeutic principle   To clear heat, eliminate toxic pathogen, clear blood heat and promote blood circulation.   .

Principal acupoint   **Bāxié(EX – UE9)**.

Supplemental acupoints   Ashi acupoint (tender spot). The plum – blossom acupuncture may be applied over the skin lesion. The points **Fèidiǎn** and **Qiántóudiǎn** may be chozen for patients with headache, fever and chillness due to attack of wind and heat pathogens; the bleeding therapy may be applied at **Shíxuān(EX – UE11)** for patients with much toxic heat pathogen to clear heat; **Láogōng (PC8)** and **Shàofǔ(HT8)** may be used to treat the patients with blood heat and blood stasis to clear blood heat and promote blood circulation; **Sānjiāodiǎn** and **Yángchí**(SJ4) may be used to treat patients with fever, chest distress and distension of upper abdomen due to attack of dampness pathogen.

Cautions

1) The ruptured skin lesion with infection should be treated in time.

2) The patients are restricted in bed with involved limb elevated and they should drink much water.

3) The thin paste of Jinhuang Powder mixed with honey or water is repeatedly applied over the skin lesion after the paste applied on the lesion is dry. The dressing is not necessary.

Scapulohumeral Periarthritis

Scapulohumeral periarthritis is a disease of shoulder joint with limitation of movement due to widespread adhesion of joint capsule and its surrounding soft tissues. It is more common in patients over 50 years of age.

Etiology and Pathogenesis

Scapulohumeral periarthritis often occurs in old women around the age of 50, which is also called "shoulders of the old" or "shoulders of fifties". Since it is very often caused by traumata or by the pathogenic factors of wind, coldness or dampness, it is called in traditional Chinese medicine "jianning" (restricted movement of shoulder), "loujian feng" (omalgia) or "dongjie jian" (congealed shoulder).

This disease may be produced by such causes as weak constitution of people over 50, overworking, invasion of evil wind, cold and dampness, overdue duration of fixation after a trauma. All of this will lead to chronic inflammation of the peripheral soft tissues around the shoulder, extensive adhesion, and restricted movement of the shoulder joint.

In traditional Chinese medicine, the liver stores blood and controls tendons; the spleen is in charge of digestion and controls limbs; and the kidney can store essence, control bones and produce bone marrow. If the vital energy is deficient, the external wind, cold and dampness pathogens may attack the body and block the circulation of qi in meridians; the overfatigue and muscular strain may cause stasis of blood; the invasion of wind and heat pathogens into meridians may scorch the meridians to block the circulation of qi and blood; and the phlegm and dampness pathogen may also block the meridians to cause this disease.

Main Points of Diagnosis

1. It often occurs in old women around fifty.

2. At the initial stage, there is a pain in the shoulder, which may be aching pain, dull pain or stabbing pain. In the case of a sudden occurrence the pain may be severe, with the upper arm and the elbow involved. Or there may be nocturnal pain.

3. Severe restriction of shoulder movement, even unable to do daily washing, combing and dressing at the advanced

stage. There is atrophy of the muscles in the shoulder with one or two sensitive tender points, for instance, under the acromion or in the anterior part of the shoulder. Both active and passive movements of the shoulder joint are limited, especially abduction, external rotation and elevation.

4. Long course of disease, ranging from a few months to 1 − 2 years, with possible natural cure in some cases in spite of such sequelae as muscular atrophy of the shoulder area and even stiff shoulder joint due to long − term illness.

Differential Diagnosis and Treatment

Clinical manifestation   The shoulder pain is diffuse and the tender spots are located not only on the great tuberosity of humerus bone. The soreness and pain of shoulder is worse at night and the arm is limited to raise up, laterally rotate, backward extend and abduct with difficulty to comb hair and to put a hand on the opposite shoulder. The movement of shoulder joint may cause marked muscular spasm. Following the progress of disease, the limitation of movement is worsened, but the pain of shoulder may be alleviated. At the late stage, the movement of shoulder joint is badly impaired with severe limitation to all directions. In patients caused by wind and dampness pathogens, the tongue coating is thin and white and the pulse is floating and moderate; in patients caused by cold and dampness pathogens, the tongue proper is

pale with thin and white coating and the pulse is wiry and
tense; and in patients caused by wind and heat pathogens,
the tongue proper is red with thin and yellow coating and the
pulse is floating and rapid.

Therapeutic principle   To expel wind and cold
pathogens, warm meridians and release stasis in collaterals.

Principal acupoint **Jiāndiǎn**.

Supplemental acupoints   **Hòuxī (SI3)**, **Hégǔ (LI4)**,
Nèiguān(PC6).

The reducing technique is applied to **Jiāndiǎn**; the balanced reinforce − reducing technique is applied to **Hòuxī**
(SI3).

Maneuver Therapy

(1) The patient sits on a stool. The operator stands on
the affected side of the patient and (1) fixes the wrist of the
affected limb with one hand, and performs such maneuvers
as tracing, shaking, rocking and rotating.

(2) Place the thumb, forefinger and middle finger of
the other hand on the patient's affected shoulder, thumb on
the anterior aspect and the other two fingers on the posteri-
or, to perform pinching and pressing − kneading. The per-
formance of each hand must be well coordinated with that of
the other; the exertion of strength as well as the range of
movement should be gradually increased until the patient's

shoulder is fully invigorated. Then the affected upper limb should be made to raise up, abduct, rotate laterally, adduct, extend backwardly and rotate medially.

Lumbago

7. Lumbago is a symptom with pain of waist present in many diseases. Here is the discussion of lumbago caused by attack of external pathogens and internal injury alone.

Etiology and Pathogenesis

The waist is a part of body closely related to kidney. It is also related to Jueyin, Shaoyin, Taiyang, Yinqiao, Yangqiao, Yinwei and Yangwei meridians. The etiological factors can be divided into external pathogens and internal injury. The internal injury contains the deficiency of Yang qi and deficiency of kidney to warm meridians; and indulgence of sexual behavior and depletion of kidney essence to nouish meridians. The external pathogens contain the attack of wind, cold and dampness pathogens to waist to block the meridians; the invasion of dampness after living in a damp environment for a long time; and injury due to stagnation of qi and blood caused by falling down, acute sprain or lifting heavy substance of overload.

Differential Diagnosis and Treatment

1) Wind, cold and dampness type

The patients may suffer from coldness and pain of waist, gradually aggravated and worse in cloudy and rainy days and difficulaty to move and rotate waist. The tongue coating is white and greasy and the pulse is deep, slow and moderate.

Therapeutic principle　　To expel wind and cold pathogens and eliminate dampness.

Principal acupoints　**Yāotòngdiǎn(EX – UE7)**.

Supplemental acupoints　**Hòuxī(SI3), Jǐzhùdiǎn**.

The warm acupuncture is applied to **Jǐzhùdiǎn**.

2) Deficiency of kidney type

The patients may suffer from soreness and weakness of waist and leg, worse after tiredness but relievable after lying down or by applying pressure. The patients may have spasm of lower abdomen, cold limbs, pale tongue proper and deep and thready pulse; or annoyance, insomnia, dryness in mouth and throat, flushed face, hotness in palms and soles, red tongue proper with scanty coating and wiry, thready and rapid pulse.

Therapeutic principle　To tonify kidney qi and nourish

meridians.

Principal acupoint   **Yángchí(SJ4)**.

Supplemental acupoints   **Yāotòngdiǎn (EX − UE7)**, **Sānjiāodiǎn, Shèndiǎn**.

3) Stagnation of qi and blood type

The patients may suffer from limitation of movement of waist and severe lumbago and refuse to palpate their waist. The tongue proper is dark with ecchymoses and the pulse is wiry and uneven.

Therapeutic principle   To promote circulation of blood, regulate circulation of qi and release stasis of blood.

Principal acupoint   **Hòuxī(SI3)**.

Supplemental acupoints   **Sānjiāodiǎn, Nèiguān(PC6)**.

4) Acute sprain of waist

The patients may suffer from severe lumbago caused by acute muscular sprain due to improper physical exertion in inadequate posture, limitation of movement and difficulty to stand and walk, worse during walking, coughing and sneezing. The tongue proper is red with thin and white coating and the pulse is wiry.

Therapeutic principle   To promote circulation of qi and blood, relax muscles and improve movement of joints.

Principal acupoint   **Yāotòngdiǎn(EX − UE7)**.

Supplemental acupoints   **Hòuxī(SI3), Shàozé(SI1)**. The technique of fighting between dragon and tiger is applied to **Yāotòngdiǎn(EX − UE7)**.

Raynaud's Disease

Raynaud's disease is commonly seen in young and middle-aged women and usually affecting the upper limbs but less involving the lower one, this disease is due to over excitement or cold stimulus and manifested by symmetrical and paroxysmal sudden pallor of the finger or toe followed by light purple, hectic and sensation of pain and numbness.

Etiology and Pathogenesis

Failure of the tendons to be nourished by blood due to insufficiency of the liver — yin resulting from stagnation of the liver — qi results in numbness and spasm of the limbs. Deficiency of qi and blood due to stagnation of qi and shortage of blood leads to pale fingers. Absence of enough heat due to yang — deficiency of the spleen and kidney is responsible for very cold hands and feet. Accumulation of cold, yin pathogen, in the channels causes grayish purple extremities of the limbs. Incoordination between ying and wei and debility of wei — qi give rise to hectic skin. Blood stasis is due to stagnation of qi, obstruction is due to blood stasis, and pain is due to obstruction. Inability of the tendons and vessels to be nourished due to stagnation of qi and blood brings about withered skin, myophagism and even ulcer. In short, insufficiency of the liver — yin, yang — deficiency of the spleen and kidney and stagnation of qi and blood are the original causes of this disease, while exogenous cold, the external pathogenic factor.

Main Symptoms and Signs

After sudden anger or rage, the skin of fingers or toes symmetrically and paroxysmally becomes pale, greyish purple and finally hectic and then returns to normal, which is accompanied by cold, numbness and dysesthesia of the finger which are relieved by warmth but aggravated by cold, and distending thin smaller pointed extremity of the limb with dry skin and myophagism or superficial small ulcers in severe cases, with the arterial pulse of the affected limb being normal.

Differential Diagnosis and Treatment

1) Deficiency of spleen and kidney Yang

The patients may suffer from pale complexion, cold body and limbs, fear of coldness, soreness and weakness of waist and knee, long stream of clear urine and passage of loose stool. After the attack of coldness, the terminals of limbs may turn extremely cold and the skin of fingers and toes becomes pale or cyanotic with numbness and pain. The tongue proper is pale with thin and white coating and the pulse is deep and thready.

Therapeutic principle To warm spleen and tonify kidney.

Principal acupoint **Pídiǎn** and **Shèndiǎn**.

Supplemental acupoints **Bāxié(EX – UE9)**, **Nèiguān (PC6)** and **Hégǔ(LI4)**.

The gentle moxibustion may be applied to **Bāxié(EX – UE9)** for 30 min; the moxibustion with aconite may be applied to **Pídiǎn** and **Shèndiǎn** with moxa cones in a size of a pit of date and changed for 3 – 5 times. The decoction of Cangzhu (atractylodes rhizome) 20 gm, Guizhi (cinammon twig) 25 gm, Fuzi (aconite daughter root) 10 gm, dry ginger 15 gm and Aiye (argyi leaf) 50 gm boiled in 2500 ml of water for steaming and then washing the termials of limbs, which may also be soaked in the warm decoction for 30 – 60 min, twice a day.

2) Attack of violent cold pathogen

The terminals of limbs are cold and pale or pink in color, induced by attack of coldness. The symptoms are more remarkable during cold season and the patients are afraid of coldness. The tongue proper is pale with white coating and the pulse is deep and slow.

Therapeutic principle   To expel cold pathogen and warm meridians.

Principal acupoints **Shàofǔ(HT8)** and **Mìngméndiǎn**.

Supplemental acupoints   **Bāxié (EX – UE9)** and **Xīndiǎn**.

The gentle moxibustion is applied to **Shàofǔ(HT8)** and **Mìngméndiǎn**; after acupuncture, the sparrow – pecking moxibustion is applied to **Bāxié(EX – UE9)** for 5 – 10 min. The decoction of fresh ginger 20 gm, green onion 30 gm, Fuzi (aconite daughter root) 25 gm and Aiye (argyi leaf) 50, boiled in 2500 ml of water to steam and then wash the limbs, which may also be soaked in the warm decoction for 30 min, 2 – 3 times a day.

3) Stagnation of qi and blood

The terminals of limbs may be persistently cool and cyanotic with severe pain and distention and the fingers and toes are swollen with stasis of blood. The tongue proper is dark brown with petechiae and ecchymoses and the pulse is uneven.

Therapeutic principle   To adjust circulation of qi and promote circulation of blood.

Principal acupoint **Bāxié(EX – UE9)**.

Supplemental acupoints **Gāndiǎn, Hégǔ(LI4)**.

After acupuncture, the gentle moxibustion is applied to **Bāxié(EX - UE9)** for 30 min; and the reducing technique is applied to **Gāndiǎn** and **Hégǔ** (**LI4**). The decoction of Chuanwu (aconite root) 10 gm, Caowu (wild aconite root) 10 gm, Cangzhu (atractylodes rhizome) 15 gm, Duhuo (pubescent angelica root) 15 gm, Fangfeng (saposhnikovia root) 15 gm, Liujinu (mugwort) 15 gm, Honghua (safflower) 15 gm, Guizhi (cinammon twig) 12 gm, Huajiao (prickly ash) 12 gm, Tougucao (speranskia) 20 gm and Aiye (argyi leaf) 50 gm may be used to steam and wash the limbs, 2 - 3 times a day.

4) Accumulation of damp - heat pathogen

The fingers and toes are swollen, hot and flushed or purple in color with pain, ulcer or gangrene and the patients may also suffer from dryness in mouth and dark urine. The tongue proper is red with thin and yellow coating and the pulse is rolling and rapid.

Therapeutic principle   To eliminate dampness and clear heat.

Principal acupoint   **Láogōng(PC8)**.

Supplemental acupoints   **Sānjiāodiǎn, Xiǎochángdiǎn**.

The bleeding therapy may be applied to **Shíxuān(EX - UE11)**; the reducing technique is applid to **Sānjiāodiǎn** and **Xiǎochángdiǎn**; and the Ruyi Jinhuang Powder may be externally applied to the lesions.

Chapter Three
Diseases of
Eye, Ear, Nose, Throat and Tooth

Myopia

Myopia refers to a condition in which the visual images come to a focus in front of the retina of the eye because of defects in the refractive media of the eye or of abnormal length of the eyeball resulting especially in defective vision of distant objects. It is a common disease of eyes in youths with clear near vision but poor remote vision.

Etiology and Pathogenesis

The liver stores blood and the eyes can see clearly if the supply of blood to eyes is sufficient. As the eyes are used to read and watch over a long time, the blood in eyes may be exhausted. The patients may develop myopia if the blood in eyes can not be fully replenished. The basic cause of myopia is to read and write in an improper posture with the books very close to the eyes and in a poor light.

Differential Diagnosis and Treatment

Clinical manifestation: The patients suffer from gradually impaired vision, pain and distension of eyes, dizziness, pain and distension of head and lumbago. The tongue is red and the pulse is thready.

Therapeutic principle   To tonify liver and kidney.

Principal acupoints   **Gāndiǎn** and **Shèndiǎn**.

Supplemental   acupoints   **Qiántóudiǎn,   Nèiguān** (**PC6**).

Nyctalopia

Nyctalopia, or night blindness, is a disease of eyes with normal vision in the day and poor vision at night.

Etiology and Pathogenesis

The liver can store blood and the eyes are its external orifice; and the kidney can store essence and control pupils. The eyes can see clear, if enough blood and essence can be supplied to them. Otherwise, the eyes can not see clear, if the liver and kidney are deficient to supply enough blood and essence to them. If the spleen and stomach are dificient and weak and they can not digest food and water to supply e-nough nutrients, the patients may also develop

Differential Diagnosis and Treatment

Clinical manifestation

The patients may suffer from dizziness, occasional vertigo, dryness in mouth and blurred vision or blindness at night or in dark environment. The tongue proper is red with scanty coating and the pulse is wiry and thready.

Therapeutic principle   To tonify liver and kidney.

Principal acupoint   **Qiántóudiǎn**.

Supplemental acupoints   **Gāndiǎn, Shèndiǎn**.

The reinforcing technique is applied to **Gāndiǎn** and **Shèndiǎn**; and the decoction of liver of chicken and bat's feces can be administered orally.

Glaucoma

Glaucoma is a kind of syndrome characterized by the increase in intraocular pressure leading to the injury of visual function. It can be classified into three main types: primary glaucoma, secondary glaucoma and congenital glaucoma. The primary and congenital types involve both eyes while the secondary one occurs mainly in one eye. Primary glaucoma is further divided into open – angle type and angel closure type. In traditional Chinese medicine, glaucoma corresponds to Wūfēng Nèizhàng included in disorders of the pupil, that is, Lùfēng Nèizhàng, Qīngfēng Nèizhàng, Chìfēng Nèizhàng, Hēifēng Nèizhàng and Huángfēng Nèizhàng. Among them, Lùfēng Nèizhàng and Qīngfēng Nèizhàng are more commonly seen in clinical practice and will be dealt with in this part.

Acute Angle Closure Glaucoma

Acute angle closure glaucoma (Acute congestive glauco

ma), usually found in old females, involves both eyes, but at first it may just affect one eye. The interval between the occurrences of syndromes of the two eyes is irregular. The attack is usually caused by mental depression or overwork. Clinically, it is characterized by acute increase in intraocular pressure, mixed congestion of the eyeball, corneal edema, mydriasis, greenish – blue pupil margin, accompanied with severe swelling of the eye, headache, nausea and so on. It belongs to the category of "Lǜfēng Nèizhàng" (green glaucoma) in traditional Chinese medicine. When it comes into the absolute stage, it belongs to the category of "Huángfēng Nèizhàng" (absolute glaucoma with cataract) in traditional Chinese medicine.

Etiology and Pathogenesis

The disease is due to long – standing stagnation of the liver Qi caused by emotional upset, which later turns into fire to attack the eyes; it may also be due to flaming of fire of the liver and gallbladder which may develop into wind – heat to attack the eyes, or due to retention of phlegm – dampness that turns into fire to attack the eyes. Besides, damage of Yin caused by overstrain may lead to hyperactivity of Yang and induce endogenous wind. When the wind goes upward to attack the eyes, the disease occurs.

Main Symptoms and Signs

There are four stages according to the progress of pathogeny. At the preclinical stage, following an emotional stress, there is mild headache distention in the eye and iridization but the symptoms may have spontaneous remission after rest. At the stage of attack, there is distending pain in the eyeball, severe headache, nausea, vomiting and sudden diminution of vision due to rapid increase of the intraocular pressure. An examination may reveal mixed congestion, corneal edema which presents ground – glass – like opacity, a shallow anterior chamber, fan – shaped iridoatrophy, mydriasis, disappearance of photoreaction, and grayish – white cloudy spots under the anterior capsule of the lens, The anterior chamber angles are closed. At the remission stage, the intraocular pressure reduces as a result of treatment, the symptoms subside; the visual function improves; congestion disappears; the cornea clears up and the anterior chamber angle reopens. But if high intraocular pressure persists, the anterior chamber may become adherent. The duration of this stage varies. At the chronic stage, an acute attacks that has not yet been timely treated, or repeated attacks, may lead to extensive adhesion of the anterior chamber angles, which results in continuous increase of the intraocular pressure, marked diminution of vision, contraction of visual field, higher ratio between the cup and the optic disc and pale color of the disc. The blood vessels are pushed to the nasal side, like bending – knees. The chamber angle becomes narrower or closed. Gradually the vision will completely lose and the disease will enter the absolute stage.

Main Points of Diagnosis

1. It is manifested as acute swelling of the eye, headache, nausea, diminution of vision and so on.

2. There is mixed congestion of the eye, corneal edema with misty opacity, opacity of aqueous humor. The anterior chamber becomes shallow. The pupil becomes enlarged and loses its normal circular contour, with the presence of green – blue reflection of light inside the pupil.

3. The eyeball becomes as hard as stone. The intraocular pressure usually comes up to more than 6 kPa, even exceeding 10 kPa.

4. If the persistent increase of the intraocular pressure fails to come down, later on complete blindness results. If the dilated pupil fails to constrict, if iris becomes discolored and the crystalline lens becomes yellow or yellowish – white in color, then it turns to the absolute glaucoma.

Acupuncture Treatment

The commonly used points are **Jīngmíng**(**BL**1), **Sìbái** (**ST**2), **Chéngqì**(**ST**1), **Qíuhòu**(**EX** – **HN**7), **Hégǔ**(**LI**4),

Tàiyáng(EX - HN5) and **Fēngchí(GB20)**. Choose four points for needling, once a day.

Another Acupuncture Therapy

Tàichōng(LR3) on both sides can be selected and stimulated with strong stimulation, with the needle retained for 20 to 40 minutes, once or twice a day.

3) Auricular Acupuncture

Search for sensitive points and use them in coordination with the points eye 1, eye 2, liver, etc. for needle - embedding or Semen Vaccariae plaster mounting until the remission of the symptoms.

4) Massage

Press and knead **Fēngchí(GB20)** for 30 minutes. Scrape the eye orbits for 30 minutes. Knead **Cuánzhú (BL2)**, **jīngmíng(BL1)** and **Tàiyáng(EX - HN5)** for 30 minutes respectively. Heat the eyes for 30 minutes. Press and knead **Hégǔ(LI4)** for 30 minutes, and knead **Tàichōng(LR3)** and **Gānshū(BL18)** for 30 minutes respectively.

Open - Angle Glaucoma

Open - angle glaucoma, which is also called Simple Glaucoma, is characterized by pathological increase of the intraocular pressure and an open anterior chamber angle. As it progresses slowly with slight symptoms, it is not easy to decoct it at the early stage. The disease is usually found in young adults, and males are affected more often than females. It corresponds to Qingfeng Neizhang in traditional Chinese medicine.

Etiology and Pathogenesis

Emotional depression of a person may cause stagnation of the liver Qi that will turn into fire. When the fire goes upward to attack the eyes, the disease occurs. Or, if a person suffers from retention of dampness due to hyperfunction of the spleen, phlegm will originate from the retention and form phlegm stagnation which will further convert into fire. When the fire moves upward to attack the eye, the disease is caused. Besides, deficiency of the liver and kidney, a condition called consumption of primordial Yin, will result in asthenic fire, and attack of the eye by the fire will lead to the Disease.

Main Symptoms and Signs

At the early stage there is almost no symptom, but slight distention feeling in the eyes, headache and iridization may occur due to overwork or emotional upset. As the disease progresses, vision diminishes and visual field shrinks gradually and blindness will occur finally. Clinical examination shows that there is no change in the anterior part of the eye. The cupping of the disc of the fundus becomes wider and deeper. The cup disc ratio is above 0.5. The blood vessels are pushed to the nasal side, some of which look like bending knees, with nerve fiber layer defect. At the late stage the optic disc is pallor and looks like a cup.

The anterior chamber angle is wide. The intraocular pressure is elevated and its undulation amplitude is large within twenty – four hours.

Differential Diagnosis and Treatment in Hand Acupuncture Therapy

1) Stagnation of liver qi

The patients may suffer from mental depression, distension of flank and costal region, pain and distension of breasts and irregular menstruation in women, migraine and dryness in mouth and throat. The tongue proper is red with yellow and dry coating and the pulse is wiry.

Therapeutic principle   To disperse liver qi and improve vision.

Principal acupoint   **Yǎndiǎn**.

Supplemental acupoints   **Shàofǔ(HT8)**, **Gāndiǎn**.

Qiántóudiǎn and **Gāndiǎn** are used to treat upward exacerbation of liver Yang with headache, vertigo, flushed face and bitter taste in mouth; **Shàoshāng(LU11)**, **Guānchōng**

(SJ1) and **Shāngyáng**(LI1) are used to treat headache, red eyes and tinnitus due to stagnation of liver with fire pathogen.

2) Deficiency of liver and kidney   The patients may suffer from emptiness and pain of head, emission, soreness of waist, tinnitus and dull pain of eyes. The tongue proper is red with thin and white coating and the pulse is thready and weak or wiry and thready. ·

Therapeutic principle   To tonify liver and kidney.

Principal acupoints   **Shèndiǎn** and **Yǎndiǎn**.

Supplemental acupoints   **Yángchí**(SJ4), **Hégǔ**(LI4), **Gāndiǎn**.

Láogōng(PC8) and **Sānjiāodiǎn** are used for poor communication between heart and kidney with insomnia.

Nervous Tinnitus

Nervous tinnitus refers to the disease characterized clinically by high – pitch tinnitus and without dysfunction in the hearing ability, and it belongs to the category of "Ěr lóng" in traditional Chinese medicine.

Etiology and Pathogenesis

It is mostly related to insufficiency of kidney – *yin* and ascension of deficient *fire* which disturb the clear orifice, or is related to deficiency and consumption of meridians around the eyes and ears, or ascension of liver *fire* which disturbs upwards the clear orifice, and causing tinnitus.

Main Symptoms and Signs

1. Continuous high – pitch tinnitus, aggravated at night.

2. Mostly, subjective tinnitus.

3. Mostly, normal hearing ability.

3. Normal or slight collapse in tympanic membrane.

Acupuncture and Moxibustion

Select 3 to 5 points from **Ěrmén** (SJ21), **Tīnggōng** (SI19), **Tīnghuì**(GB2), **Yìfēng**(SJ17), **Zhōngzhǔ**(SJ3), **Wàiguān**(SJ5), **Yánglíngquán**(GB34), **Zúsānlǐ**(ST36) and **Sānyīnjiāo**(SP6). Punctured with medium stimulation. The treatment is given once a day.

Differential Diagnosis and Treatment in Hand Acupuncture

1) Deficiency of kidney essence

The tinnitus is low and weak and the deafness becomes worse and worse. The patients may also have vertigo, soreness of waist and emission of semen. The tongue proper is red in color and the pulse is thready and rapid.

Therapeutic principle   To tonify kidney Yin.

Principal acupoints   **Sānjiāodiǎn** and **Piāntóudiǎn**.

Supplemental acupoints   **Hégǔ**(LI4), **Láogōng**(PC8), **Yángchí**(SJ4).

2) Deficiency and weakness of spleen and stomach

The patients may suffer from tinnitus, poor appetite,

weakness of limbs and passing loose stool. The tongue proper is pale with thin and white coating and the pulse is thready and weak.

Therapeutic principle   To strengthen spleen and regulate stomach.

Principal acupoints   **Mìngméndiǎn** and **Piāntóudiǎn**.

Supplemental acupoints   **Pídiǎn, Yèmén(SJ2)**.

3) Excessive fire pathogen in liver and gallbladder

The patients may have sudden onset of tinnitus, headache, flushed face, bitter taste in mouth, dryness in throat, annoyance, anger and constipation. The tongue proper is red with yellow coating and the pulse is wiry and rapid.

Therapeutic principle   To clear heat pathogen in liver and gallbladder.

Principal acupoints   **Yángchí(SJ4)** and **Piāntóudiǎn**.

Supplemental acupoints   **Hégǔ (LI4), Yèmén (SJ2),
Sānjiāodiǎn**.

Deafness

1. Senile Deafness

Senile deafness refers to the progressive decrease of hearing ability on both ears after middle age and it is often related to heredity. Clinically it is characterized by bilateral, chronic and progressive deafness, and it belongs to the category of "Shèn xū ěr lóng" (deafness due to kidney deficiency) in traditional Chinese medicine.

Etiology and Pathogenesis

Kidney opens into the ears and kidney qi flows into the ears. Only when essence and qi in the kidney are sufficient and plentiful, and when the source of bone marrow is nourished, can the hearing ability be sensitive, and can the distinguishing powder be higher. In the senile cases, essence and qi in the kidney start to subside, resulting in decrease of the hearing ability.

Main Symptoms and Signs

1. It often starts after 50 years old, the hearing ability decreases progressively, and especially hearing ability of high frequency decreases first.

2. The decrease of the hearing abilities symmetrical on both sides, diagnosed as nervous deafness without vibration.

3. The tympanic membrane looks grey, dark and lustrousless in color.

Acupuncture and Moxibustion

Select 3 to 5 points from **Ěrmén (SJ21), Tīnghuì (GB2), Yìfēng(SJ17), Zhōngzhǔ(SJ3), Wàiguān(SJ5), Yánglíngquán (GB34), Zúsānlǐ (ST36)** and **Sānyīnjiāo (SP6)**. Retain the needles for 30 minutes to one hour. The treatment is given once a day.

2. Sudden Deafness

Sudden deafness, a sensorineural hearing loss, occurs abruptly for reasons unknown. Its main clinical feature is a sudden profound sensorineural deafness, accompanied by tinnitus and dizziness and a tendency to get cured spontaneously. The disorder is usually unilateral and occurs more often in females and mostly in the middle – aged. In traditional Chinese medicine, it belongs to the category of "Bào lóng" or "Cù lóng", both meaning sudden deafness. It is elated to invasion of external pathogenic wind and internal injury of seven emotional factors, which causes stagnation of meridians in the ear orifice, disharmony between *qi* and *blood* .

Main Points of Diagnosis

1. In some cases there exist mental factors or a history of virus infection prior to the attack of the disease.

2. It occurs abruptly. The patient often has severe deafness or even loses hearing entirely within an hour or one day.

3. There is often an accompanying tinnitus or vertigo.

4. Otic endoscopy examination indicates normal.

5. Audiometric curve shows that the deafness is a sensorineural hearing loss. Low – frequency deafness and even deafness are seen more often and recruitment may be present.

Acupuncture and Moxibustion

The points are **Yìfēng (SJ17)**, **Tīnggōng (SI19)**, **Tīnghuì(GB2)**, **Ěrmén(SJ21)**, **Zhōngzhǔ(SJ3)**, **Wàiguān**

(SJ5), **Yánglíngquán**(GB34), **Xiáxī**(GB43), **Sānyīnjiāo** (**SP6**) **and Zúsānlǐ**(ST36). 3 to 4 points among them are selected each time. Reducing method. The treatment is given once daily.

Injection therapy may also be applied. 2 ml of *Danshen zhusheye* or *Danggui zhusheye* is injected into **Yìfēng**(**SJ17**) and **Tīnggōng**(**SI19**). The treatment is given once every other day, ten treatments as one course.

Differential Diagnosis and Treatment

1) Upward exacerbation of liver fire

The patients may suffer from sudden onset of tinnitus and deafness, headache, vertigo, flushed face, bitter taste in mouth, dryness in throat, annoyance, anger with worsened tinnitus and deafness. The tongue proper is red with yellow coating and the pulse is wiry and rapid.

Therapeutic principle   To clear liver fire and open orifices of sense organs.

Principal acupoints   **Nèiguān** (**PC6**) and **Zhōngzhǔ** (**SJ3**).

Supplemental acupoints   **Shèndiǎn, Gāndiǎn, Yèmén** (**SJ2**).

2) Deficiency of kidney essence

The patients suffer from tinnitus, deafness, dizziness or vertigo, soreness and weakness of waist and weakness. The tongue proper is red in color and the pulse is thready and weak.

Therapeutic principle　To tonify kidney essence and tonify Yin to suppress exacerbated Yang.

Principal acupoints　**Shèndiǎn, Sānjiāoshū(BL22).**

Supplemental acupoints　**Yángchí(SJ4), Hégǔ(LI4)** and **Yèmén(SJ2).**

3) Deficiency and weakness of spleen and stomach

The patients may suffer from tinnitus and deafness, worsened by tiredness, poor appetite, tiredness and shortness of breath. The tongue coating is thin and white and the pulse is thready.

Therapeutic principle　To tonify qi, strengthen spleen and upward transport clear Yang.

Principal acupoints　**Pídiǎn** and **Hégǔ(LI4).**

Supplemental acupoints　**Piāntóudiǎn, Sānjiāodiǎn.**

The reducing technique is used to treat excessive type of deafness; the reinforcing technique and gentle moxibustion are used to treat deficient type of deafness and the needles are retained for 20 - 30 min, once a day or every 2 days. One therapeutic course is composed of 10 times of treatment and a rest of 3 - 5 days is arranged between 2 therapeutic courses. The ear acupoint may produce a better therapeutic result.

Chronic Rhinitis

Chronic rhinitis is a chronic inflammatory change o the nasal mucosa, mainly due to the protraction of acute rhinitis. Its main symptom is nasal obstruction. This disease is called "Bí zhì" (nasal obstruction) in traditional Chinese medicine.

Etiology and Pathogenesis

It is related to *qi* deficiency of the lung and spleen which fails o protect the body from being attacked by pathogenic factors, and which leaves the evils and toxins to linger in the body, resulting in accumulation of the evils in meridians and collaterals, stagnation of *qi* and *blood* as well as nasal obstruction.

Main Symptoms and Signs

1. Intermittent, alternative or continuous nasal obstruction.

2. Swelling or hypertrophy of nasal mucosa, which is as big as mulberry fruit and in dark − red color, especially in inferior nasal concha.

Main Points of Diagnosis

1. The nasal obstruction is either alternate, intermittent or continuous.

2. The nasal mucosa swells or becomes thick, especially that of the inferior nasal concha.

3. Hyposmia is fluctuating.

4. There is pain and itching in the throat and tinnitus or hypoacusis may occur.

Differential Diagnosis and Treatment

Clinical manifestation   The patients may suffer from nasal obstruction and running nose aggravated by attack of wind and cold pathogens, increase of sticky nasal discharge, dizziness, headache, distension and pain in root of nose, continuous sneezing and profuse watery nasal discharge.

Therapeutic principle   To disperse lungs and open their orifice.

Principal acupoints   **Qiántóudiǎn** and **Fèidiǎn**.

Supplemental acupoints   **Sānjiāodiǎn, Yèmén (SJ2), Yángchí(SJ4)**.

Acute Tonsillitis

Acute tonsillitis is an acute nonspecific inflammation of the palatal tonsillae. Its clinical features are fever, headache, sore throat which is aggravated when swallowing, and reddened and swollen palatal tonsillae. It is called "Fēng rè rǔ é" or "é fēng", both referring to acute tonsillitis caused by pathogenic wind – heat.

Etiology and Pathogenesis

It is related to pathogenic wind and heat which invade through the mouth and nose to attack the lung and stomach, resulting in the condition that heat in the lung ascends and attacks the throat by the lung meridian; or related to accumulation of heat in the stomach and spleen due to preference for spicy and greasy food and further attack of pathogenic wind and heat, resulting in accumulated heat in the throat.

Main Symptoms and Signs

1. Fever around 40℃ .

2. Sore throat aggravated by swallow, even difficulty in swallow, pain radiating to the ear.

3. Redness and swelling in tonsil, purulent secretion in the opening of crypt, congestion in pharyngeal mucosa, sub-maxillary lymphadenovarix with tenderness.

Main Points of Diagnosis

1. The patient shivers with fever (the highest tempera-ture may be around 40℃) and has accompanying headache and soreness o the limbs. In infant patient convulsion may present.

2. Sore throat occurs and it may radiate to the ears. The pain becomes more severe when the patient swallows and there is even dysphagia in severe cases.

3. The palatal tonsils congest and swell or there may be yellow – white exudate on the lacunae, which in severe cases forms a false membrane that can be easily erased.

4. There may be congestion of the throat as well as red-ness and swelling of or small white dots on the retropharyn-geal lymph follicles.

5. There may be swelling and tenderness of the lymph nodes in the angle of mandible.

6. There is an increase in the number of the white blood cells and neutrophils.

7. The onset is abrupt and its duration is short. Generally it can get cured in 5 – 7 days.

Acupuncture and Moxibustion

1) Choose 2 to 3 points each time from **Hégǔ(LI4)**, **Nèitíng(ST44)**, **Qūchí(LI11)** and **Yújì(LU10)** and puncture with reducing method twice a day.

2) Use shallow puncture for blood letting. Puncture the points of **Shàoshāng(LU11)** and **Shāngyáng(LI1)** with a three – edged needle to let out blood so that pathogenic heat can be removed. Or the veins of the back of the ear are punctured to let out three to five drops of blood. If necessary, the same can be done the next day.

3) It is advisable to inject 0.5 to 1.0 ml of *Yuxingcao zhu she ye* or *Chaihu zhu she ye* into both **Píshū(BL20)** and **Qūchí(LI11)**, and the injection is given once a day.

Hand Acupuncture

Differential Diagnosis and Treatment

1) Wind and heat type
The patients may suffer from fever, sore throat, diffi-

culty to swallow, hoarseness of voice and spitting sputum and saliva. The tongue proper is red with yellow coating and the pulse is full and rapid or floating and rapid.

Therapeutic principle   To expel wind pathogen from body surface and clear heat from throat.

Principal acupoint   **Yānhóudiǎn**.

Supplemental acupoints   **Shàoshāng** (LU11), **Shāngyáng**(LI1), **Yújì**(LU10). The bleeding therapy is applied to **Shàoshāng** (LU11), **Shāngyáng** (LI1) and **Yújì** (LU10).

2) Excessive heat type

The patients may suffer from sore throat, headache, fever, foul smell from mouth, spitting yellow and sticky sputum, thirst with desire to drink much water, annoyance and passing short stream of dark urine. The tongue coating is yellow and the pulse is wiry and rapid.

Therapeutic principle   To clear heat and fire pathogen.

Principal acupoints   **Xiǎochángdiǎn** and **Yānhóudiǎn**.

Supplemental acupoints   **Hégǔ** (LI4), **Wèichángtòngdiǎn, Shāngyáng**(LI1), **Qūchí**(LI11).

3) Yin deficiency type

The patients may suffer from sore throat, dryness of mouth, hotness in heart, palms and soles, hoarseness of voice, flushed face and lips. The tongue proper is red with scanty coating and the pulse is thready and rapid.

Therapeutic principle   To enrich Yin and clear heat.

Principal acupoints **Shèndiǎn** and **Yānhóudiǎn**.

Supplemental acupoints **Láogōng** (PC8), **Shàofǔ** (HT8), **Sānjiāodiǎn**.

Odontalgia

Odontalgia, commonly called as toothache, is a symptom in oral cavity usually induced or aggravated by cold, hot, sour or sweet stimulation.

Etiology and Pathogenesis

There are many pathogenic factors to produce this symptom, but they can be divided into the deficient and excessive factors. The excessive toothache is caused by wind and fire pathogens and stomach heat. The hand and foot Yangming meridians pass through upper and lower teeth respectively. The invasion of wind and heat pathogens to the meridians or the stagnation of heat in stomach may block Yangming meridians, then the stagnated fire pathogen may flare up along meridians to cause toothache. The kidney can control bones and the teeth are the protrusion of bones. The deficiency of kidney Yin with flaring – up of deficient fire may also cause toothache of the deficient type. The indulgence of sour and sweet foot and the poor oral hygiene may produce caries and toothache.

Differential Diagnosis and Treatment

1) Excessive type

The patients may suffer from severe toothache, swollen gum, foul smell from mouth and constipation. The tongue proper is red with yellow coating and the pulse is wiry.

Therapeutic principle   To clear heat in Yangming meridians.

Principal acupoints   **Hégǔ(LI4)** and **Xīndiǎn**.

Supplemental acupoints   **Xiǎochángdiǎn** and **Sānjiān (LI3)**.

2) Deficient type

The patient may suffer from fluctuated dull toothache, loose teeth, dizziness, soreness and weakness of knee and leg, dryness in mouth and annoyance. The tongue tip is red in color and the pulse is thready or thready and rapid.

Therapeutic principle   To tonify kidney Yin.

Principal acupoint   **Shèndiǎn**.

Supplemental acupoints   **Sānjiāodiǎn** and **Yángchí (SJ4)**.

Epistaxis

Epistaxis (rhinorrhagia) is a common clinical symptom caused by many reasons and happening in various diseases. In mild cases, only nasal discharge is mixed with blood, and in severe cases it may endanger the patient's life.

The most common sites of nasal bleeding are the mucosal vessels over the cartilaginous nasal septum and the anterior tip of the inferior turbinate. Bleeding is usually due to external trauma, nose picking, nasal infection, or drying of the nasal site cannot be seen; these can cause great problems in management. If the blood drains into the pharynx and is swallowed, nosebleed may escape diagnosis. In these cases, bloody vomitus may be the first clue.

Underlying causes of nosebleed such as blood dyscrasia, hypertension, hemorrhagic disease, nasal tumors, and certain infectious diseases (measles or rheumatic fever) must be considered in any case of recurrent or profuse nosebleed without obvious causes.

In traditional Chinese medicine, the condition is termed "Bí nǜ", which simply means epistaxis, "Bí hóng" (flood – like nosebleed), "Hóng hàn" (red sweat) and is thought to be caused by dry lungs.

Etiology and Pathogenesis

The reasons of rhinorrhagia can be listed in the following:

1. **Heat Preponderance:** It indicates hat the invaded pathogenic heat mixes with internal accumulated heat and causes hyperactivity o heat in the lung and stomach, resulting in crazy circulation of blood;

2. **Reverse – flowing** qi **:** For example, frustration and anger turn the stagnation of liver qi into fire which flares and brings blood upwards, pushing blood to circulate outside of vessels;

3. **Yin Deficiency in the Lung and Kidney:** It refers to flaming – up of deficient fire which injures collaterals in the nose;

4. **Spleen Qi Deficiency:** It refers to dysfunction of spleen qi which fails to restrain *blood* to circulate inside the blood vessels, causing extravasation. Also there is nasal bleeding due to trauma, which is regarded as syndrome of blood stasis.

Main Symptoms and Signs

1. In mild case, there is bloody nasal discharge or slight nasal bleeding. In severe cases, there is gushing nasal bleeding, very often at sudden onset. The blood can flow out from the anterior nostrils and also can flow into the throat via posterior nasal nostrils. The nasal bleeding can be intermittent, recurrent and continuous and can happen in one nostril and also can happen in both nostrils.

2. There is capillarectasia or bleeding spots in the anterior part of nasal septum. In severe nasal bleeding, it is not easy to notice bleeding location, and only possible to see gushing bleeding location after cleaning away the blood in the nose. Extensive blood oozing in nasal mucosa can be noticed in recurrent cases.

Main Points of Diagnosis

1. Try to find the spot of nosebleed. Bleeding is apt to occur in the mucous membrane of Kiesselbach's area.

2. Try to analyze the causes of nosebleed. Detailed inquiry about the history of the case should be made. If possible, examinations of the nasal cavity and nasopharynx, blood text, blood pressure determination, fundus examination and other necessary checks should be done.

3. The condition depends on the location and the quan-

tity of the nosebleed. Shock may occur in severe cases. Repeated occurrence can cause anemia.

Differential Diagnosis and Treatment

1) Heat pathogen in lungs   The patients may suffer from nasal bleeding, dryness in nose and mouth and stimulating cough. The tongue proper is red and the pulse is rapid.

Therapeutic principle   To clear heat pathogen in lungs.

Principal acupoint   **Fèidiǎn**.

Supplemental acupoints   **KǒngZùi (LU6)** and **Qiántóudiǎn**.

2) Heat pathogen in stomach

The patients may suffer from nasal bleeding, dryness in nose, thirst with desire to drink water and foul smell from mouth. The tongue proper is red with yellow coating and the pulse is full and rapid.

Therapeutic principle   To clear heat pathogen in blood.

Principal acupoint   **Dàchángdiǎn**.

Supplemental acupoints   **Sānjiāodiǎn, Shàoshāng (LU11), Fèidiǎn** and **Qiántóudiǎn**.

3) Heat pathogen in liver

The patients may suffer from nasal bleeding, headache, vertigo, red eyes, dryness in mouth and bad temperment. The tongue proper is red with yellow coating and the pulse is wiry and rapid.

Therapeutic principle   To clear liver fire.

Principal acupoint   **Gāndiǎn**.

Supplemental acupoints   **Fèidiǎn, Pídiǎn,** and **Nèiguān(PC6)**.

Other External Treatment

In the case with active nasal bleeding, it is necessary to stop bleeding first with various hemostatic methods external- ly in accordance with the principle of "to deal with symptoms in acute condition", and then to identify types of diseases and offer related treatment. The commonly − used hemostatic methods for external treatment are listed as follows.

1) Hemostasis

(1) Cold compress: This is to put towel soaked in cold water or ice − bag on the patient's forehead, neck, or the acupoint **Yǎmén(DU15)**. The neck is the site where *Yang- ming meridians, du channel* and *taiyang meridians* go through, cold compress on the neck is able to restrain *yang*, subside fire for cooling blood and stopping bleeding.

(2) Finger pressing: Insert some aseptic cotton coated with *Powder of puff − ball* or *Yunnan white drug − powder* onto the anteroinferior area of nasal septum, then press the nasal wings with the forefingers to stop the bleeding.

(3) Nose − blowing method: This is to take a little *Crinis Carbonisatus, Powder of Lasiosphaera seu Calvatia,*

Baicao shuang, *Yunnan white powder* and blow into the bleeding location of the nose, several times a day till bleeding stops.

(4) Nose – stuffing method: This is to pound *Herba A-grimoniae*, *Herba Cephalanoploris* and *Herba Ecliptae* to take juice as oral medication, and also able to smash these herbs to stuff the nose.

(5) Plugging: When the above – mentioned methods prove ineffective, the method of plugging either the anterior naris or the posterior naris can be used.

2) Leading Blood Downwards

Repeated occurrence of nosebleed marked by small amount of blood are mostly the result of the injury of blood vessels caused by the upward flow of deficiency – fire. *Powder of Evodia Fruit* can be applied on the sole; or warm water can be used to wash the feet so as to guide the ascending fire downwards; or the paste of *Bulbus Allii* is to be applied onto the acupoint **Yǒngquán**(**KI**1) which also help to stop the bleeding.

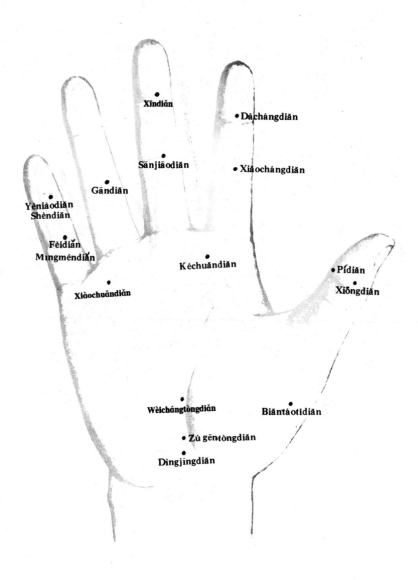

Xīndiǎn

Dàchángdiǎn

Sānjiāodiǎn

Xiǎochángdiǎn

Gāndiǎn

Yèniàodiǎn
Shèndiǎn

Fèidiǎn
Mìngméndiǎn

Kéchuǎndiǎn

Pídiǎn

Xiōngdiǎn

Xiàochuǎndiǎn

Wèichángtòngdiǎn

Biǎntáotǐdiǎn

Zú gēntòngdiǎn

Dìngjīngdiǎn

249

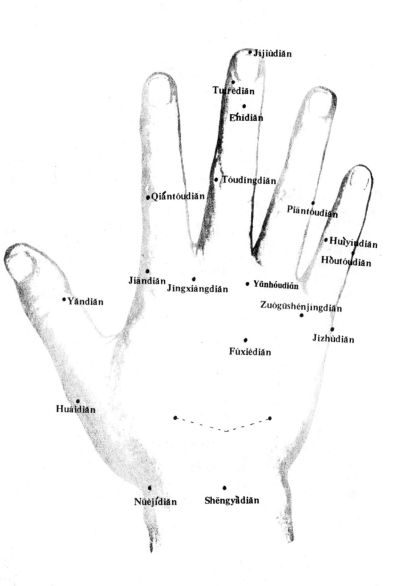

Jíjiùdiǎn

Tuīrèdiǎn

Éhidiǎn

Tóudǐngdiǎn

Qiántóudiǎn

Piàntóudiǎn

Huìyīndiǎn

Hòutóudiǎn

Jiāndiǎn

Jǐngxiàngdiǎn

Yānhóudiǎn

Yǎndiǎn

Zuógǔshénjīngdiǎn

Jǐzhùdiǎn

Fùxièdiǎn

Huáidiǎn

Nüèjídiǎn

Shēngyàdiǎn

图书在版编目(CIP)数据

手针疗法:英文/赵昕主编;

乔晋琳,李国华编辑 －北京:学苑出版社,1997.11

ISBN7－5077－1375－X

Ⅰ.中… Ⅱ.①赵… ②乔… ③李…

Ⅲ.手针足针疗法－英文 Ⅳ.R245.32

中国版本图书馆 CIP 数据核字(97)第 20139 号

手针疗法

赵昕 主编

乔晋琳,李国华 编

学苑出版社出版

(中国北京万寿路西街 11 号)

邮政编码 100036

北京大兴沙窝店印刷厂印刷

中国国际图书贸易总公司发行

(中国北京车公庄西路 35 号)

北京邮政信箱第 399 号 邮政编码 100044

英文版 32 开本

1997 年 11 月第 1 版第 1 次印刷

ISBN7－5077－1375－X

05200

14－E－3133P